54467A

2000
996B

Dora Hsi-Chih Chao, M.D.

Physician and Assistant Director, Blue Bird
Clinic, Methodist Hospital, and Assistant Professor of Pediatrics and Neurology, Baylor University College of Medicine, Houston

Ralph Druckman, M.D.

Neurologist, Blue Bird Clinic, Methodist
Hospital, and Assistant Professor, Departments
of Neurology and Physiology, Baylor University
College of Medicine, Houston

Peter Kellaway, A.M., Ph.D.

Director, Blue Bird Clinic, Methodist Hospital,
and Associate Professor, Department of Physiology, Baylor University College of Medicine,
Houston

Convulsive Disorders of Children

W. B. SAUNDERS COMPANY

Philadelphia and London   1958

Preface

THIS BOOK is a revised version of a manual on convulsive disorders which the authors originally prepared for the use of residents in the Blue Bird Circle Children's Clinic. It is an attempt to provide a concise and simple review of diagnosis, treatment and management of the convulsive disorders and is based primarily on the data collected and developed in the Clinic since its establishment in 1949.

The emphasis is clinical, but sufficient physiology and pathology are given to afford the reader an understanding of the fundamental mechanisms involved.

Without wishing to involve them in the responsibility for the shortcomings of this book, we would like to express our appreciation for the suggestions made by friends and colleagues who read and criticized the book in its original version. We would like to acknowledge particularly the many constructive changes suggested by Sir Charles Symonds, Dr. Arthur Ward, Mr. Joe Pennybacker, F.R.C.S., and Dr. Samuel C. Little. Most of these suggestions have been incorporated in the present volume.

PETER KELLAWAY

Blue Bird Clinic

Contents

CHAPTER I

Introduction

THE EARLIEST known references to epilepsy occur in early Greek writings. The very term *epilepsy* had its origin in the Greek words meaning "to lay upon" or "to seize," and the implication was that some supernatural influence had taken control of the patient. This idea that the epileptic is a person possessed or stricken by supernatural forces has persisted to some extent even to the present day.

Hippocrates recognized that epileptic seizures had natural causes and that these primarily affected the brain; however, ignorance and superstition concerning epilepsy persisted because of the dramatic and often bizarre character of its various manifestations. These attitudes continue to be reflected in public prejudice against epileptics and in the shame because of the seizures felt by many patients and their families. Only recently have significant steps been taken to rectify discriminatory and irrational legislation which reflects these prejudices and misconceptions.

The problem is not a minor one, for the incidence of "convulsive" disorders is high. About 4 per cent of children have a seizure at one time or another in their lives, if only in association with fever. Statistics of the armed forces indicate that in the 18 to 20 year age group, about 1 in every 200 of the male population is subject to a convulsive disorder. No accurate information is available concerning

1

the incidence of epilepsy in older age groups, but the evidence suggests that it is considerably higher in children than in adults.

Epilepsy is a symptom and not a disease, and classification of the epilepsies has suffered because of the frequent difficulty in establishing definite etiology. As a result, classification has tended to become largely description and in terms of seizure character, rather than in terms of etiology. Another factor which has interfered with the development of knowledge of epilepsy is the frequent use of a single term with multiple and varying meanings. Improved methods of investigation developed in the last half century, however, have provided increasing information about the causes of epilepsy. Roentgenology, including pneumoencephalography and angiography, has provided an invaluable tool for the detection and localization of structural abnormality of the brain. The rapid growth of electroencephalography in the past 20 years has been the most significant development in the field, frequently providing objective evidence of disturbed cerebral function where all other tests are unrevealing. The development of these modern methods of studying brain structure and function in the living patient has made possible new insight into the nature and origin of "convulsive" disorders. Long term studies with the new techniques should eventually provide a coherent and complete picture of these disorders and make possible a rational and consistent clinical classification with reliable criteria for diagnosis and prognosis.

The present problems in this field are:

(1) Uniform definitions of various seizure types, so that results of various investigators can be correlated.

(2) Long term study of each variety of epilepsy by means of combined clinical and laboratory studies, in order to determine the natural history of each type.

(3) Further investigation as to the etiology of various seizure states, including viral studies and studies of allergic and toxic factors.

(4) Development of more effective therapeutic measures, both medical and surgical.

(5) Dissemination of knowledge concerning epilepsy to the general public, to industry and to the law maker, so that the discrimination against patients with epilepsy will be eliminated.

Definitions

The term *epilepsy* covers such a wide range of phenomena that its definition has varied. Clinically, it may be defined as a condition characterized by transient and usually recurrent episodes of change in consciousness or experience, without an obvious, immediately precipitating extracerebral cause, such as head injury or intoxication. To be defined as epilepsy, these symptoms should result from sudden, spontaneous, excessive and transient neuronal discharge, occurring either focally or diffusely in the brain. The manifestations of epilepsy are quite varied and range from subjective tingling in a limb or abdominal distress, to loss of consciousness with or without convulsive movements. The evidence of the abnormal ganglionic discharge may be represented in the electroencephalogram by abnormal electrical activity; however, because of the limitations of electroencephalography, the absence of electrographic abnormality does not rule out the diagnosis of epilepsy.

There are terms with narrower meanings which are used in the field of epilepsy. The word *seizure* refers to any single epileptic attack and is synonymous with *fit*. *Convulsion* is a term which indicates a prominent motor or muscular component in an epileptic attack. Such convulsions may be generalized and involve most of the striated musculature, or they may be focal and limited to the muscles of one limb or even of a single muscle group.

Petit mal is a term used with many different meanings. Some use it to refer to any seizure which does not proceed to a generalized convulsion. Others limit its use to lapse, myoclonic and akinetic attacks, while still others limit its scope to only the lapse attacks. *Grand mal* universally means generalized convulsion. *Psychomotor* attacks are those in which the patient performs semipurposeful, coordinated movements, such as buttoning clothes or walking from one place to another, without consciousness of these activities. Some use the term psychomotor to indicate automatisms of temporal lobe origin, while others, making no such limitations, use it to include automatisms of frontal or diencephalic origin.

Classification

The disadvantages of a classification of the epilepsies into petit mal, grand mal and psychomotor attacks are several. There is no uniformly accepted definition of petit mal, so that ambiguity and confusion result from its use. Furthermore, this classification is purely descriptive and gives no indication of etiology, even when the cause may be known. Because the foregoing classification is the one in common usage, it is necessary to know how each term is used in order to relate it to pathophysiological entities.

Epilepsy is not a disease entity but a symptom or sign of disturbed cerebral physiology. The pattern of the seizure is determined by the localization of cerebral abnormality, and this abnormality may be the result of a wide variety of causes. The ideal classification should include:

(1) Adequate description of the seizure pattern.
(2) Localization of the causative cerebral abnormality.
(3) Etiology of the cerebral abnormality.
(4) Evaluation of the functional efficiency of the patient. This necessitates the assessment of the relative roles of: (a) loss of cerebral tissue, and (b) impairment of function of the remaining brain by abnormal neuronal discharge.

It should be recognized that though it is not always possible to determine all of the foregoing features, every effort should be made to evaluate the patient fully in these terms.

The classification of the convulsive disorders which follows is essentially etiological. These disorders are:

(1) Idiopathic (or genetic) epilepsy.
(2) Symptomatic epilepsy.
(3) Conditions related to or confused with epilepsy (such as benign febrile convulsions and breath holding).

Idiopathic epilepsy refers to a specific convulsive disorder in which no anatomical lesion of the brain has been demonstrated and in which genetic determinants are important. Only the following types of seizure, as specifically defined later, may be of idiopathic origin:

(1) Lapse or absence attacks.
(2) Myoclonic jerks.
(3) Akinetic attacks.
(4) Automatisms.
(5) Generalized convulsions.

Symptomatic seizures are those resulting from a lesion of the brain. Indications of this lesion and its location may be provided by examination of the nervous system or by any of the various laboratory procedures, such as roentgenology and electroencephalography. The seizures may be classified as arising from one epileptogenic focus (unifocal), from multiple foci (multifocal) or from diffuse cerebral disease. The foci may be cortical or subcortical (usually diencephalic). The history and the results of special tests may reveal the cause and localization of the cerebral lesion. Seizures of all types, with the possible exception of the classical absence variety, may occur in symptomatic epilepsy.

Conditions which are related to or which may be confused with epilepsy are those disorders in which there are convulsive attacks, but in which there is a necessary and invariable extracerebral accessory factor. Such conditions include convulsions due to excessive fever, hypoglycemia, toxins and anoxia. The causative agent *transiently* upsets cerebral function in such a way as to produce excessive neuronal discharge, which becomes clinically evident as a convulsion. Breath-holding spells, febrile convulsions and Stokes-Adams attacks are of this kind.

REFERENCES
1. Temkin, O.: The Falling Sickness. Baltimore, Johns Hopkins Press, 1945.
2. Lennox, W. G.: Science and Seizures. New York, Harper and Brothers, 1946.
3. Fabing, H. D.: Epilepsy and the law. M. Clin. North America, 42:361, 1958.
4. Jasper, H. and Kershman, J.: Electroencephalographic classification of the epilepsies. Arch. Neurol. and Psychiat., 45:903, 1941.
5. McNaughton, F. L.: The classification of the epilepsies. Epilepsia, 1:1, 1952.
6. Williams, D.: Modern views on the classification of epilepsy. Brit. M. J., 1:661, 1958.

CHAPTER 2

The Basis of Seizure Manifestations

Functional Anatomy

Knowledge of the normal functions of various regions of the brain facilitates the localization of the site of origin of a seizure. Much information has been gathered about the functions of the different regions of the cerebral cortex through animal experiments, by correlation of seizure patterns with the site of lesions demonstrated at autopsy or surgery and by electrical stimulation of the surface of the cerebral cortex in humans operated upon under local anesthesia. The latter technique makes it possible to obtain subjective reports of the particular experiences of the patient when various discrete regions of the brain are stimulated.

LOCALIZATION OF FUNCTION IN THE CEREBRAL CORTEX

Stimulation of a localized area in the intermediate frontal region produces turning of the *eyes* to the opposite side. Excitation of the frontal adversive field anterior and superior to the eye area produces turning of the *eyes, head and body* to the opposite side (fig. 1). The cortical representation of areas producing different body movements has been mapped out by stimulation of the precentral gyrus, or motor strip, in man. Leg movements are produced by stimulation

7

LOCALIZATION OF
SEIZURE MANIFESTATIONS

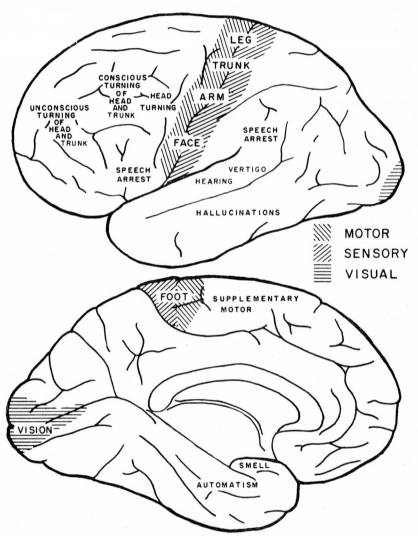

Figure 1. The general regions from which various seizure phenomena arise. The lateral aspect of the brain is depicted in the upper drawing; the mesial aspect of the left cerebral hemisphere is depicted in the lower drawing.

close to the sagittal fissure near the midline. Lateral to this are the areas producing movements of the trunk, and more inferiorly, in the precentral gyrus, those producing movements of the upper limb and face. Inferiorly, vocalization of crude sounds is produced in the region representing control of the lips and tongue.

The area of representation of a body part is proportional to the extent and variety of use to which that part is put in a given species. Thus, for example, the area controlling the hand in humans is much greater than that controlling the abdomen. This disparity is a reflection of the complexity of connections necessary to produce the varied movements of which the hand is capable, as compared to the limited movements of the larger abdominal musculature. The excitability of the areas of representation is directly proportional to their extent; hence, the larger the area of representation of a given body part, the greater its excitability. This fact has clinical importance in that such areas are much more likely to be involved in a local epileptogenic discharge; therefore, focal epilepsy beginning in the hand or face is much more likely to occur than are seizures involving body parts with lesser cortical representation, such as the neck or thigh.

Within the longitudinal fissure, just anterior to the area representing movements of the leg, lies a region which has been called the *supplementary motor area.* Stimulation here produces movement of the contralateral hand upwards, and the head and eyes of the patient move so that they face the palm of the uplifted hand. Crude vocalization or, conversely, arrest of speech may also result from stimulation in this region.

Electrical stimulation of the postcentral gyrus usually produces a sensation of tingling or of numbness on the opposite side of the body. There is a sequence of sensory representation in the postcentral gyrus similar to the motor sequence in the precentral gyrus. Thus the lower limb is represented superiorly, the upper limb more laterally and the face inferiorly. A second sensory area lies in the downward extension of the postcentral gyrus into the sylvian fissure. Both sides of the body are represented in the *second sensory area,* with a slight predominance of the contralateral side.

Excitation of the occipital lobe results in a subjective sensation of bright lights, often colored, which may seem to be moving. The things seen on stimulation here are unformed objects rather than visual hallucinations. Excitation of the occipital lobe also may result in an interference with vision described as blurring, clouding or even loss of sight.

Electrical stimulation of the temporal lobe has produced a variety of changes. Since the cortical control of hearing and of the vestibular apparatus lies in the superior temporal gyrus, stimulation here produces sensations of crude sound (noise, buzzing) and of vertigo. The elicited sound is usually referred to the opposite ear. Stimulation of the uncal region has produced olfactory sensations, usually of an unpleasant character. Stimulation of the insular region has resulted in sensations of taste and also in abdominal discomfort.

Patients with temporal lobe foci may have psychic experiences elicited by local electrical stimulation. They may remember scenes from the past, revisualize previous experiences and hear songs which may continue as long as the electrical stimulus is applied. Fear, also, has occasionally resulted from stimulation of the anterior temporal region.

Automatic behavior has resulted from stimulation of the mesial aspect of the temporal lobe. Such automatism in spontaneous seizures usually involves stereotyped and well coordinated movements, such as searching, fumbling with clothes, dressing or undressing. These occur without the patient being able to recall them afterward.

Perceptual distortions occur with excitation of the temporal lobe, so that the patient may think things are farther away or closer to him or larger or smaller than they are in actuality. At times the patients realize that their perceptions are incorrect, and this results in a dissociated state which might be mistaken for a purely functional disorder. Thus ictal psychic, perceptual and behavioral alterations are the common manifestations of discharging lesions of the temporal lobe.

Arrest of speech may be produced by stimulation of a number of regions. These include an inferior frontal zone just anterior to the area of representation of facial movement in the precentral gyrus, another just anterior to the foot area on the mesial aspect of the hemisphere, and a third region where the parietal and temporal lobes meet (fig. 1). These effects are generally elicited from the dominant hemisphere, and in each case the aphasic difficulty arises from an inability to recall the correct words rather than from an inability to articulate. Stimulation of the inferior precentral gyrus, where lip and tongue movements are represented, produces in either hemisphere an arrest of speech because of an inability to articulate, akin to paralysis of the vocal apparatus. The patient retains his ability to think of the words.

Autonomic responses also may be elicited from the cerebral cortex. Salivation is produced from the rolandic region just above the sylvian fissure. Stimulation of the insula produces nausea, abdominal sensations and borborygmi. Pallor and flushing have resulted from insular stimulation. Changes in respiration occur on stimulation of the tip of the temporal lobe and the orbitofrontal region. Changes in pupillary size may result from stimulation of the supplementary motor, cingulate and peristriate cortex.

MANIFESTATIONS OF DISCHARGE IN SUBCORTICAL STRUCTURES

Experimentally, the hypothalamus has been demonstrated to have a marked influence on autonomic function. There is also evidence that it exerts an influence on postural mechanisms and on behavior. Ictal hypothalamic discharge can produce vasomotor changes resulting in pallor, flushing and alterations in blood pressure. Changes in gastrointestinal motility also may occur. Rage attacks are thought to have a hypothalamic origin and most autonomic and pain attacks (equivalents) are believed to originate in diencephalic structures.

Although the experimental evidence is meager, lapse, myoclonic and akinetic attacks and massive spasms are thought to arise in subcortical structures, probably the brain stem.

Histopathology of Brain Scars

Cortical scars are the commonest causes of symptomatic epilepsy. There are several different types of epileptogenic scars. After a cerebral laceration with penetration of the dura or in a drained cerebral abscess one may find a scar with dense adhesions between the dura and pia or between the dura and brain (meningocerebral cicatrix). These adhesions carry blood vessels and collagenous fibers into the brain.

Local cortical ischemia at birth or late in life may also result in scarring. The ischemia produces local death of nerve cells and results in regional convolutional atrophy, so-called microgyria.

Occlusion of a cerebral artery or an intracerebral hemorrhage may be followed by resorption of the destroyed tissue with resultant cyst formation. Gliosis occurs around the cyst, and in this region areas of abnormal discharge may be created.

The typical cerebral scar has a central zone in which no nerve cells survive. Surrounding this is an intermediate zone in which there are islands of nerve cells. This region peripherally merges into the surrounding normal brain. In the intermediate zone there is a slow and progressive neuronal destruction, and there is evidence that this process may continue for years. Here small regions show acute swelling of the oligodendroglia, fragmentation of the processes of the protoplasmic astrocytes (astrocytic clasmatodendrosis) and fat-filled phagocytes. There is a reduction in the total number of neurons in this zone, and the remaining nerve cells show chromatolysis. Here, too, the number of precapillary and capillary vessels is greatly reduced.

The source of the focal epileptogenic discharge is to be found in the intermediate zone. The degenerating nerve cells are believed to be more excitable (possibly because of inadequate blood supply) and to discharge excessively and hypersynchronously. When this discharge becomes of sufficient intensity, a clinical seizure results. In patients with seizures caused by tumors, interference with the blood supply of the remaining nerve cells by the presence of the tumor possibly provides a mechanism for seizure production. The tumor itself is not a source of any discharge.

Depth Recording

Much basic information essential to the understanding of the physiology of epilepsy has been obtained by the use of electrodes implanted into the brains of epileptic patients. Information is thus gathered about the electrical activity of buried cortical and subcortical structures during periods of seeming normality, as well as at the heights of seizure activity. Striking abnormality may occur in the buried structures, while a simultaneous scalp recording shows nothing remarkable. In periods when the patient shows no clinical sign of abnormality, there may be bursts of localized discharge occurring in the depths of his brain. Such abnormal electrical activity may be almost continuous, depending upon the area involved, without any overt manifestation of seizure-like character. However, subtle changes in the patient's affect and personality have been shown to be associated with these episodes.

The abnormal electrical activity may spread locally, or at other times more diffusely, to produce generalized hypersynchronous activation of both cortical and subcortical structures. The character and degree of the clinical manifestations are directly related to the rate and degree of this spread.

REFERENCES

1. Penfield, W. and Rasmussen, T.: The Cerebral Cortex of Man: A Clinical Study of Localization of Function. New York, The Macmillan Co., 1950.
2. Penfield, W. and Jasper, H.: Epilepsy and the Functional Anatomy of the Human Brain. Boston, Little, Brown and Co., 1954.
3. Spielmeyer, W.: The anatomic substratum of the convulsive state. Arch Neurol. and Psychiat., 23:869, 1930.
4. Foerster, O. and Penfield, W.: The structural basis of traumatic epilepsy and results of radical operation. Brain, 53:99, 1930.
5. Zimmerman, H. M.: The histopathology of convulsive disorders in children. J. Pediat., 13:859, 1938.
6. Penfield, W. and Humphreys, S.: Epileptogenic lesions of the brain; a histologic study. Arch. Neurol. and Psychiat., 43:240, 1940.

CHAPTER 3

Sequence of Events in a Seizure

FOR SEVERAL hours or even days before an attack, some patients may become irritable, anxious, tired, depressed or mentally dull. This phase, which is known as the prodrome, is correlated with an increase of abnormal activity in the electroencephalogram.

Frequently, the onset of the actual seizure is preceded by a sudden subjective change which the patient recognizes as a warning of an impending seizure. These sensations, which are similar from attack to attack for a given patient, are referred to as the aura, and may consist of a rising epigastric sensation or other subjective experience. Actually, the aura differs from the seizure proper only in the fact that the effect of the aura is evident only to the patient himself. The aura is a manifestation of the beginning of the abnormal neuronal discharge (which is the basis of the seizure), at a time when this discharge remains highly localized and has not attained a very great magnitude. Physiologically, the difference is only a quantitative one; clinically, the difference is that the aura is subjective and the seizure proper is overt or objective. It is now well established that the aura and even the prodrome may occur without being fol-

15

lowed by an overt attack. The development of an overt seizure depends upon whether or not the build-up of the abnormal discharge attains a certain magnitude or spread.

The spread of the discharge determines the clinical sequence of events. An involvement of the motor system gives rise to tonic and clonic spasms of the skeletal musculature; the spread to certain specific areas of integration gives rise to changes in or loss of consciousness; the activation of autonomic centers gives rise to changes in respiration, urination and defecation and to excessive salivation. Invariably, if the spread is sufficient to produce a generalized seizure, there is complete loss of consciousness.

With diminution of the neuronal discharge, the clinical manifestations of the seizure stop. Depending upon the character, the duration and the severity of the clinical seizure, the patient may then go into a stage in which there is evidence of impaired mental and physical function. This has been called the *postictal state*. It may consist of a period of confusion or stupor, or the patient may fall into a deep sleep. Immediately following a seizure the patient may have generalized weakness, fatigue or headache. In exceptional cases the patient may feel better after an attack.

Certain neurological abnormalities may be present in the postictal period. These may have localizing significance in terms of the site of origin of the epileptic discharge and hence of the underlying lesion. A transient postictal hemiparesis, aphasia or even a persistent unilateral reflex change may point to the presence of a focal cerebral epileptogenic lesion.

It should be pointed out that all the possible phases of an epileptic seizure may not be present. Prodromes are relatively uncommon. The aura is often present and its character may have important localizing significance. Generalized seizures are almost invariably followed by a postictal phase, the intensity of which is usually proportional to the severity of the attack.

The following description illustrates all the phases of a generalized seizure: The patient is noted to become irritable for several hours or days (prodrome). He himself may not recognize this change in his behavior. He then develops a mildly unpleasant epigastric sensation which persists for several seconds (aura), until he suddenly becomes rigid in extension, unconscious and apneic. He falls to the floor and urinates, and after a short period in a state of tonic extension develops a generalized clonic jerking of the body and extremities. The clonic jerking gradually becomes less frequent and diminishes in intensity until it finally ceases. The patient then is comatose and flaccid, and his respiration is labored. Slowly, consciousness returns, but the patient may be stuporous or confused for a variable period (postictal phase) before returning to the pre-seizure state.

Initiation of a Seizure

Seizures may begin in many different ways. They may start with clonic movements of a part, such as the hand, with a turning of the head, eyes or body to one side or with posturing movements. More complex activities, such as chewing, swallowing or puckering movements of the mouth, are other common seizure phenomena. In psychomotor seizures, complex, semipurposeful movements, such as fumbling with the clothes, may be performed. Conversely, inhibition of movement or of postural tone or an inability to speak may be the initial phenomenon of a seizure.

Paresthesias (commonly, numbness and tingling in a part of the body), hallucinatory episodes of a visual, auditory, olfactory or gustatory type or disturbances of vision, such as blurring or scotoma, may be the initial phenomena of an attack. Impairment of consciousness or complete loss of consciousness are common initial phenomena in seizures.

Perceptual illusions may initiate an attack, or indeed constitute the primary or major feature of a seizure. Objects may appear larger or smaller than they actually are or sounds may seem louder or more distant than in reality. Similarly, the patient may have psychic or subjective experiences of an inappropriate nature: familiar surroundings may appear unfamiliar or strange ones seem familiar. Persistent memories or thoughts may crowd into consciousness, or the patient may experience unprovoked fear, anxiety or vague unpleasantness.

The character of the phenomenon which constitutes the initial feature of a seizure is dependent upon the part of the brain which is first involved by the seizure discharge. The variations in seizure type are primarily then a reflection of the localization of function in the brain, and therefore have clinical value in localizing the origin of discharge and the causal lesion. For example, a seizure which begins with a movement of the left index finger may be presumed to have its origin in the area representing that movement in the right precentral gyrus. As the seizure develops, more of the brain is involved in the epileptic discharge, and once the seizure has become generalized, nothing of localizing value may be detected. However, the presence of a generalized seizure does not preclude the possibility of its having a focal origin. Seizures which arise focally in the cerebral cortex may spread so rapidly or involve so quickly the subcortical structures, that they give rise to nothing but generalized attacks. Even if there are localizing features to an attack, these may be missed by the observer or forgotten by the patient postictally. Thus, the absence of focal features in seizures does not eliminate the possibility of focal cerebral origin of the attacks.

Precipitants of Seizures

Seizures may be precipitated by many factors. Fever is a common precipitant in children. Emotional disturbances, fatigue and hyperventilation, which may occur naturally in exercise, are common precipitants. Sleep often brings on seizures, particularly those of temporal lobe origin. Bright light or interrupted light is a precipitant of lapse attacks. A seizure may be brought on by a specific movement, or by a specific sensory stimulus (reflex epilepsy). Music, sometimes of a quite specific nature, may bring on attacks, the so-called "musicogenic epilepsy." Seizures of the massive spasm variety (pp. 45–50) have many precipitants, including noise, handling, feeding and the states just prior to and after sleep.

Excessive hydration, either from excessive fluid intake or from certain metabolic disturbances which occur in pregnancy or menstruation, is a potent activator of seizures. Alcohol, both directly and indirectly through a water-loading effect, is also a common precipitant.

Conversely, patients often report that they can inhibit or abort their seizures by carrying out some particular procedure, such as rubbing the involved part. Concentrated attention will decrease the number of attacks experienced by patients with lapse attacks.

CHAPTER 4

Symptomatic Epilepsy

A SEIZURE may be produced in any living being if certain conditions prevail. Thus a normal individual can be caused to have a convulsion under conditions such as excessive hydration, excessive heat or by the action of certain chemical agents such as Metrazol.

The tendency to have spontaneous seizures, called *epilepsy,* can be the result of either genetic or acquired factors or a combination of the two. In genetic epilepsy, seizures arise due to an inborn exaggeration of the normal potentiality for the development of seizure activity, without any lesion of the brain. When anatomic abnormality of the brain is present and is the cause of the seizures, the epilepsy is said to be *symptomatic.*

Any lesion which affects the nerve cells of the cerebrum may produce seizures. Such lesions may involve the brain diffusely or involve only a very localized part of it, and they may be due to trauma, anoxia or ischemia, infection, tumors, toxic factors or degenerative processes. The incidence of the various etiological factors in the production of epilepsy varies with age. At birth cerebral anoxia and trauma are major causes of injury to the brain and thus of resultant seizures. In the early years of life infections of the meninges and brain are the common causes of brain damage, while in young adult life trauma assumes more importance. In the middle years of life tumors are more frequent causes of seizures, whereas in late life ischemic cerebral lesions secondary to atherosclerosis are the most frequent causes of epilepsy. There is much overlapping of these etio-

19

logical agents in the various age groups. The degenerative disorders (cerebral lipoidoses and presenile dementias) are rare but possible causes of epilepsy.

Each of these etiological conditions has a natural history of its own, the seizures being one of many features which change with time. Widespread severe damage to the brain is most often produced by anoxia, encephalitis and toxic factors (for example, acute lead encephalopathy). The diffuse disturbance of cerebral function determines the clinical features, such as delirium, convulsions and coma. If the disturbance is sufficiently severe, the patient may die in the acute phase. With lesser damage the patient may recover, the amount of recovery being inversely proportional to the severity of the original injury to the brain. A number of nerve cells of the brain may die and the remaining neurons integrate their activities anew. The loss of many cortical neurons may be reflected in persisting intellectual deficit and spasticity. There may be partial recovery, with scattered regions of the cerebral cortex containing nerve cells which continue to live in an abnormal nutritional state. These neurons continue to function, but in a hyperirritable fashion. Such abnormal collections of nerve cells constitute "epileptogenic foci." There may be many residual foci or possibly just one such focus. A "ripening" is apparently necessary for such foci to become epileptogenic and, as a consequence, years may elapse from the time of the cerebral injury to the appearance of seizures. Discharging foci may develop at different times in different parts of the damaged brain. They also may become spontaneously inactive at different times. These phenomena have been falsely interpreted as a "migration" of the lesion from one part of the brain to another.

The electroencephalogram reflects the changes in the underlying brain. In the acute phase of diffuse cerebral disorder, the EEG shows generalized slow abnormality and possibly various types of paroxysmal or focal abnormality. With recovery, the EEG may revert to normal, but one or more foci of abnormal discharge may appear with the "ripening" of epileptogenic areas. Such electrographic abnormality may appear without clinically evident seizures.

The severity, extent and acuteness of the disease process will determine the clinical picture, including the convulsive aspects of the clinical presentation. To illustrate, a child may have a mild meningoencephalitis with several convulsions in the acute phase of this illness, and yet recover completely from the illness with no apparent residual deficit. If the recovery from the acute illness is incomplete, the patient may be left with some mental retardation, motor defect or recurrent convulsions. Toxic conditions, such as lead encephalopathy, may produce severe diffuse brain damage in the acute phase. Seizures are more common in this acute phase, but they may also occur more chronically if there is incomplete recovery from the brain damage due to the acute intoxication. The ultimate prognosis in patients with tumors of the brain depends upon the nature of the tumor and not upon the associated seizures. If a cerebral glioblastoma is the cause of the seizures, medication may easily control the convulsive manifestations, yet in all probability the patient will die in spite of attempts at surgical excision of the neoplasm. When seizures result from a scarring of the brain secondary to a penetrating injury of the skull, chronic epilepsy may be the only evidence of persisting abnormality of the brain. In degenerative disorders, such as the cerebral lipoidoses, recurrent seizures are merely one aspect of a clinical picture which includes a gradual deterioration of intellect, vision and motor function, all of which continue till the death of the patient.

Symptomatic epilepsy may be a reflection of diffuse cerebral abnormality, of a localized epileptogenic lesion, of multiple epileptogenic lesions or of both a diffuse and focal abnormality. The subdivision of symptomatic seizures into diffuse and focal groups is an aid in determining the etiology and thus the treatment and prognosis of the seizure state.

The pattern of seizure frequently provides an indication of whether the underlying cerebral disorder is diffuse or focal. Myoclonus, that is small scattered jerks occurring synchronously or asynchronously in various parts of the body, is almost pathognomonic of diffuse cerebral dysfunction. Akinetic, head-nodding and massive spasm attacks are common patterns of seizures in diffuse encephalopathies. A child with diffuse cerebral damage may have seizures of many types, including generalized, focal, akinetic and massive spasm attacks. The electroencephalogram is of great help in deciding whether the underlying cerebral disorder is diffuse or focal.

Focal epilepsy occurs when there is a single circumscribed lesion of the brain (unifocal), or when there is activity of several separate epileptogenic lesions (multifocal). Unifocal epilepsy is manifest in recurrent seizures which are all essentially of the same character, that is, all of them have a similar pattern of onset. Difficulty in differentiating unifocal from multifocal epilepsy may arise when the focus causing the seizure is in a clinically silent area. In such instances, the seizure manifestations become obvious only when other more expressive regions of the brain become involved in the spread of the seizure discharges. If this spread always follows the same pathways, the seizures will appear to come from just one focus. If the spread varies in its direction from time to time, then the seizure manifestations vary and the observer may falsely conclude that more than one focus exists.

The presence of a single focus of epileptogenic discharge as indicated by recurrent seizures of similar pattern suggests an underlying scar of the brain, possibly consequent upon remote trauma, or, less commonly, a small neoplasm. Abnormalities on examination and laboratory testing, as well as detailed history, will help to establish the etiology of the seizures more certainly.

Variation in the pattern of attack from one seizure to another is suggestive though not conclusive evidence of more than one epileptogenic lesion. Multifocal epilepsy is most commonly the end result of remote diffuse injury to the brain, regardless of whether such damage was of infectious, toxic, anoxic or traumatic origin. A large tumor involving the brain may disturb the function of more than one region of the cerebral cortex at the junction of normal brain with the tumor. Thus, in its early phases a tumor may produce unifocal epilepsy, and later, when the tumor is much larger, it may give rise to multifocal seizures. For example, in the case of a widespread tumor in the region of the left central sulcus, one type of seizure may begin with movements of the right index finger, while in the same patient other attacks may begin with numbness of the right side of the face.

The distinction between single focal and multifocal lesions is somewhat academic as long as the foci are fairly close to one another. The distinction between unifocal and multifocal seizures is of greater clinical significance when the foci are widely separated in one hemisphere or when independent foci exist in both cerebral hemispheres. The decision as to whether single or multiple epileptogenic lesions exist is one which must be made before cortical resection is carried out for the treatment of epilepsy. Similarly, hemispherectomy is not likely to improve the seizure state when active epileptogenic foci exist in both cerebral hemispheres.

CHAPTER 5

Symptomatic Seizures of Childhood

MODERN studies have clearly shown that, contrary to the classic concept, the vast majority of seizures in childhood are of symptomatic origin. Combined electrographic and clinical studies have shown that relatively few children with seizures have idiopathic epilepsy. A surprising number are found to have discharging electrical foci of a type generally associated with static or atrophic cortical lesions (scars or microgyria). Other types of electrographic findings which are now established as evidence of brain damage are much more common than are electrical patterns associated with idiopathic epilepsy.

Clinically, as our knowledge of seizure patterns has developed, more and more cases of epilepsy are being classified as symptomatic. The symptomatic nature of a seizure often may be established merely by recognizing the significance of certain features of the attack. These features may be quite momentary and seeming unremarkable, yet be most revealing if their significance is recognized. The presence of neurological abnormality is, of course, important in establishing a diagnosis of symptomatic epilepsy, but it is becoming increasingly clear that the absence of neurological findings does not necessarily

23

rule out such a diagnosis. More than 50 per cent of the children with focal seizures and discharging electrographic foci show no other evidence of neurological abnormality.

Similarly, a history of cerebral insult contributes to the diagnosis of symptomatic epilepsy, but a failure to find in the history any evidence for a cerebral injury should not be considered to weigh too strongly against this possibility. A large percentage of patients with definite clinical and electrographic evidence of focal or diffuse "brain injury" do not have a history which clearly establishes either the nature or time of the cerebral insult. The causes of symptomatic seizures in childhood are many and diverse. The main etiological agents are listed below in relative order of incidence:

(1) Birth injury and anoxia.

(2) Inflammatory lesions of the brain, such as meningoencephalitis, exanthemata with cerebral involvement, postimmunization encephalopathy or focal cerebritis (abscess).

(3) Vascular accidents, such as dehydration with phlebothrombosis or arterial occlusion with infarction.

(4) Head injury.

(5) Congenital malformations.

(6) Brain damage secondary to prolonged febrile seizures.

(7) Toxic encephalopathy (*e.g.*, lead or thallium).

(8) Cerebral tumors.

(9) Degenerative and metabolic cerebral disorders (*e.g.*, lipoidoses or phenylketonuria).

(10) Parasites (*e.g.*, toxoplasmosis or cysticercosis).

1. Birth Injury and Anoxia

Damage to the brain during the birth process is probably the most common cause of seizures in childhood. If there is cephalopelvic disproportion (contracted pelvis or rigid soft parts), the excessive moulding of the head may cause lacerations of the cerebral venous system or compression of cerebral arteries against the tentorium, with resulting cerebral infarction. Precipitate labor and difficult forceps delivery increase the possibility of injuries of this type.

Prematurity predisposes to cerebral damage because of the unusual vulnerability of the immature brain to all types of insult.

Excessive narcosis and anesthesia are significant causes of fetal anoxia and the subsequent development of seizures in infancy or childhood. Also, not uncommonly, seizures develop in children as a result of anoxia consequent to prolapse of the cord, to premature separation of the placenta or to prolonged and difficult labor.

The early signs of cerebral birth injury include pallid asphyxia, poor respiration, episodes of apnea, poor sucking, absence of the Moro reflex, rigidity and retraction of the head, strabismus, pupillary inequalities and convulsions. Later indications of brain damage include spastic hemiplegia or monoplegia, congenital diplegia, mental defect and microcephaly. These gross signs of cerebral birth injury are easily recognized, but there are other less dramatic signs which point to brain damage of lesser severity. Excessive sleepiness or sleeplessness, irritability, unexplained vomiting and delayed developmental milestones in the young infant, and hyperactivity and short attention span in the older child, may all be signs of milder degrees of damage.

2. Inflammatory Lesions of the Brain

Seizures are frequently the result of cerebral infection. The attacks may occur in the acute phase of the infection or appear months or years later. The seizures of the acute phase reflect the great disturbance in cerebral metabolism resulting from the infection, while the later attacks reflect the epileptogenic activity of damaged neurons which survive the acute infection. Meningoencephalitis, encephalitis accompanying exanthemata, primary viral encephalitis, postinoculation encephalopathy and focal cerebritis may produce diffuse or focal epileptogenic lesions.

MENINGITIS

Infections which are primarily meningeal often affect the adjacent cerebral tissue. This effect is partly "toxic" and partly caused by thrombosis of superficial cortical veins. Damage of this type may occur in acute pyogenic meningitis (meningococcal, influenzal, streptococcal or pneumococcal), and also in more chronic forms of meningeal infection (tuberculosis, syphilis or torulosis). While with proper management many cases make complete recoveries, failure to discover and treat such infections early and effectively often results in the development of chronic epilepsy.

ENCEPHALITIS

Encephalitic involvement with exanthemata has recently been shown to occur far more frequently than was previously suspected. Electroencephalographic studies have provided objective evidence of this fact. Serial EEG studies have shown that the diffuse cerebral disturbance of the acute phase may resolve and leave only a discrete epileptogenic focus. Clinical seizures may not develop until months or years after the acute illness.

Measles (rubeola) and chickenpox (varicella) are the exanthemata most commonly associated with an encephalitic component, but German measles (rubella) may rarely produce a cerebral inflammation. Nonexanthematous infectious diseases of childhood, such as mumps and pertussis, may also have an associated encephalitic component.

Seizures commonly accompany the viral encephalitides, and chronic epilepsy is a fairly common residual of this type of infection.

POSTIMMUNIZATION ENCEPHALOPATHY

Active immunization involves a minor risk of a "hypersensitivity" reaction. Such reactions often affect the nervous system, particularly when the inoculation is for rabies, pertussis or smallpox. Histologically these reactions produce perivenous inflammation with demyelination. Clinically the acute manifestations are confusion, irritability, stupor, delirium, coma and convulsions. Chronic seizures of various types, with or without other evidence of brain damage, may persist after recovery from the acute phase of the illness.

FOCAL CEREBRITIS (BRAIN ABSCESS)

A localized inflammation of the brain may develop through a direct spread of infection from infected sinuses or from an infected middle ear. The temporal lobe is involved in the ear infections while the frontal lobe may be affected in a frontal sinusitis.

Seizures and a discharging electrical focus are indicative of such a development. Early treatment of the infection by drainage and antibiotics may lead to rapid healing, but, if treatment is ineffective, the focal cerebritis may become encapsulated (abscess) and require surgical excision. If healing results in scar formation, the scar may have a surrounding epileptogenic region which may become the source of seizures years later.

3. Vascular Accidents (Dehydration with Phlebothrombosis, Arterial Occlusion with Infarction)

The development of cerebral venous thrombosis is a significant complication of vomiting, diarrhea and other illnesses of infancy associated with severe dehydration and marasmus. If the thrombosis is extensive and involves smaller cerebral veins, there may be enough interference with the circulation of the brain to produce transient or even permanent brain damage, with resultant seizures and other indications of cerebral dysfunction. The degree of dehydration and toxemia resulting from the systemic disease determines the likelihood of such vascular complications.

Thrombosis of cerebral arteries, while not as common as in adults, does occur in children. Dehydration and toxemia are the usual causes of this type of vascular accident.

Cerebral embolisms may occur in bacterial endocarditis and in congenital heart disease of the type in which there are septal defects. They may also occur as a complication of cardiac catheterization. The resulting cerebral infarct may be a source of seizures both in the acute phase and later after the development of a residual cortical scar.

4. Head Injury

Closed head injury may produce brain damage as a result of concussion or focal contusion. Similarly, penetrating injuries produce brain damage as a result of direct laceration or by secondary infection. It is not uncommon in children for seizures to result from what appeared to be relatively mild head injuries.

Seizures may occur immediately or years after a head injury. Often head injury is implicated as the cause of an initial seizure because the patient was observed to fall and, when picked up, was unconscious. In many such instances, however, this is a mistaken diagnosis, for the fall was merely the initial event in a first seizure of other etiology.

5. Congenital Malformations

The time of gestation is probably a much more significant period for the possible occurrence of brain insult than is generally realized.

Growth and differentiation of the fertilized egg follow a definite sequential pattern. Noxious influences of various types may impede growth or differentiation or both, and once a developmental stage is interrupted, there may be no further opportunity later in development for completion of the missing or incomplete stage. Thus, noxious influences, which in adult life might have only a very transient effect upon cerebral function, may leave permanent residua if allowed to operate upon the developing fetus.

It has been well established that anoxia, infection and certain genetic defects may, during intra-uterine life, alter the normal course of development. Fetal anoxia may be suspected when there is a history of uterine bleeding or when the mother has had surgery requiring general anesthesia, especially during early pregnancy.

Certain maternal infections also have a damaging effect upon the developing fetus. German measles is the most common offender. A majority of infants whose mothers had German measles in the first two months of pregnancy have congenital malformations. Syphilis and toxoplasmosis are other infections which may pass the placental barrier and interfere with normal fetal development.

Certain diseases associated with seizures are of primary genetic origin. Tuberous sclerosis and phenylketonuria are two examples. Secondary genetic changes may be induced by roentgen ray irradiation, and this most commonly occurs when the mother is exposed to fairly high doses of roentgen rays during early pregnancy. It is clear that there must be many factors other than those mentioned above which may operate in utero to produce congenital dysplasias.

The character and degree of the congenital abnormalities produced by these various agents depend in large part upon the stage of fetal development attained at the time the noxious influence is active. For example, rubella produces malformations of the brain, ears, eyes and heart if it occurs within the first trimester of pregnancy, but it apparently produces no significant change in any structure if it occurs after this critical period.

Implication of congenital malformation as the cause underlying a seizure disorder is suggested when other indications of congenital defect, such as dysplastic facies or structural anomalies of the heart, kidneys, eyes or ears, are present. A family history of similar defects may also be considered suggestive evidence for this type of diagnosis, as also may be a history of difficulty in maintaining the pregnancy.

The classical neurocutaneous dysplasias, such as tuberous sclerosis, Sturge-Weber syndrome and the congenital defects associated with German measles and mongolism, are easily recognized. However, less obvious cases of congenital developmental defect in which mental retardation, seizures and dysplastic features are the only findings are much more common. In these the recognition of anomalies as minor as epicanthal folds may be important in making the diagnosis.

6. Brain Damage Secondary to Prolonged Febrile Seizures

The great majority of children with benign febrile convulsions do not suffer any resultant brain damage. Rarely, if a febrile seizure is prolonged, severe and associated with much cyanosis, brain damage may result. The exact mechanism by which this is brought about is uncertain, but increased metabolic demand in excess of nutritional supply, resulting from seizure activity, fever and anoxemia, probably represents the main cause of such cerebral damage. Another possible mechanism is a localized vascular occlusion occurring during the convulsion. Once brain injury has occurred in such seizures, the evidence indicates that the damaged region may subsequently serve as a source of epileptogenic discharge with consequent epilepsy.

7. Toxic Encephalopathy

Toxic encephalopathy may result from such conditions as heavy metal intoxication (lead and thallium), ingestion of organic phosphates (chlordane) or aromatic substances (naphthalene or camphorated oil), or an excessive intake of salicylates. Seizures may occur immediately after the intake or chronically, if there is permanent damage after resolution of the acute encephalopathy.

8. Cerebral Tumors

Intracranial neoplasms in childhood mainly originate in the cerebellum and brain stem, and less often involve the cerebral hemispheres. Tumors of the cerebellum and brain stem do not give rise to epileptic discharge, and seizures are not part of their usual clinical presentation. Although cerebral tumors are a rare cause of seizures in childhood, the presence of such lesions must be given serious consideration in patients who have seizures and associated *progressive* functional deficit, such as increasing hemiparesis. Certainly a seizure patient who is found to have papilledema should be considered a tumor suspect.

9. Degenerative and Metabolic Disorders

Degenerative cerebral disorders are a rare cause of seizures of childhood. The cerebral lipoidoses, such as Tay-Sachs disease, are the most common degenerative disorders of the central nervous system in childhood. Progressive mental deterioration, impaired vision and increasing motor defect occurring in association with epilepsy suggest the possibility of this type of disease.

The nerve cells of the brain are the ones primarily involved in these lipoid diseases, and seizures are frequent. Occasionally in demyelinating processes such as Schilder's disease there may be an extension of the pathological change from the white matter to the cortical and deep gray matter with resultant seizures.

10. Parasitic Involvement of the Brain

Cerebral involvement by parasites is a very rare cause of seizures in this country. Infection with toxoplasmosis may occur in utero or postnatally, resulting in gross brain damage, chorioretinitis, hydrocephalus, seizures and scattered cerebral calcifications.

Cysticercosis involving the brain is quite rare in the United States and Canada; it is more common where public health facilities are not of a high order. Acutely, the patients present with seizures and indications of increased intracranial pressure. Later the cerebral cysticerci may calcify and be evident on skull roentgenograms. The clinical features in the chronic phase are those of multifocal epilepsy.

Malaria, hydatid cysts, schistosomiasis and trypanosomiasis may involve the brain and cause seizures, but these are rarely seen here.

11. Other Causes

Special causes of cerebral disturbance, which may be reflected in seizures, include transient epileptogenic encephalopathy, kernicterus and subacute inclusion body encephalitis. Transient epileptogenic encephalopathy is a syndrome in which a child who previously developed normally develops seizures of various types, progressive mental deterioration and often spasticity and weakness. The seizures are re-fractory to anticonvulsant medication and the course is generally a downhill one, reminiscent of the cerebral lipoidoses or subacute inclusion body encephalitis for which the syndrome may be mistaken. However, after several months or even years there is a spontaneous change for the better. The seizures lessen in severity and frequency; the mentality and motor coordination improve. The child may become quite normal again, but there may be some residual mental dullness. The cause of this syndrome is uncertain, and it is possible that these patients suffer from a subacute encephalitis of undetermined cause.

In kernicterus the excess bile salts have a toxic action on the nerve cells of the brain. The neuronal damage may be reflected in mental retardation, spasticity, choreo-athetosis and occasionally in chronic recurrent seizures. The seizures may not appear for months or years after birth.

Subacute inclusion body encephalitis is a cerebral disorder of suspected viral cause. The clinical features include seizures of various types, mental and motor deterioration and a gradually downhill course over several months until death.

Clinical Correlations: Localization and Etiology
UNIFOCAL SEIZURES

If all attacks have the same pattern and particularly if they begin with clearly recognizable focal features, such as isolated jerking of an extremity, the assumption is that a single epileptogenic lesion is responsible. The presence of abnormal neurological signs, the localization of which correlates well with the suspected location of the discharging lesion, provides strong supportive evidence for the existence of a circumscribed epileptogenic lesion. If the attacks are thought to originate from a single focus, it is then necessary to try to establish the exact localization and, most important, the nature of the lesion.

Electroencephalography is the simplest and most productive laboratory procedure for localizing epileptogenic lesions. It may also throw some light on the nature of the lesion (chapter 14). Roentgenology, including air studies and angiography, may provide further information on the localization and nature of the lesion, but its usefulness is limited primarily to neoplasms and other gross structural changes.

EXAMPLE: *Temporal Lesion*
        A.W., Clinic No. B-548

This girl of 8 years was delivered by elective cesarean section and weighed 8 pounds 12 ounces at birth. When she was 6 weeks old she was dropped and her head struck a concrete floor. She was unconscious for 5 to 10 minutes. She developed normally and was well until 7 6/12 years of age, when she was found one morning limp, making chewing movements, her head rolling about, her eyes rolled back and her face ashen in color. She remained unconscious for about one minute. Six weeks later she had a further spell in the early morning, witnessed by her mother who noted that the patient was pale, lying prone and making rocking movements of her body, gagging sounds and chewing movements. The patient was drowsy after this episode.

At 7 10/12 years she began to have another type of attack. During these attacks she felt as though she were floating on air. Then one side of her face became paralyzed and she drooled out of that side. She was able to think of words but was unable to speak for the one or two minutes of these attacks.

At 7 9/12 years an electroencephalogram at another hospital was reported to have demonstrated a spike and slow wave focus in her left temporal region. There was no family history of seizures.

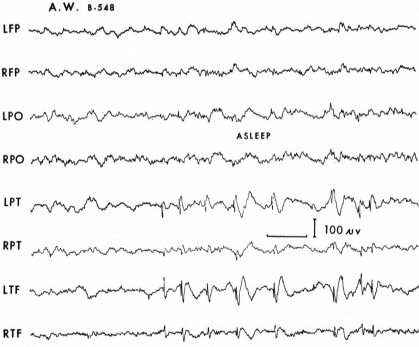

Figure 2. The repeated spike discharges, originating in the region of the left temporal electrode, are evident. There is some secondary spread of this abnormal discharge to the right temporal lead.

Before being seen at 8 6/12 years, the patient had three more spells; in the last one there was jerking of her right arm and leg.

Clinical examination at 8 6/12 years revealed no abnormality. Laboratory examinations other than electroencephalography were negative. The EEG showed a very active focus of slow-spike and spike and wave activity in the left anterior temporal region. This abnormality was thought suggestive of a discharging atrophic cortical lesion (fig. 2).

The patient was placed on small doses of Dilantin and had a further attack in which there was vomiting and postictal difficulty in speaking. The dosage was increased. Two months later she had another attack in which her mother found her semiconscious in bed. She tried to raise her head from the pillow and fumbled with her nightgown. Her eyes rolled up and she became limp for about two minutes. Mesantoin was added to the medication. She continued to have occasional attacks in sleep, during which saliva drooled from the right side of her mouth. The dosage of Mesantoin was increased. A repeat electrogram at 9 1/12 years showed no change.

Mysoline was substituted for Mesantoin but attacks continued at intervals of two to three months. The spells came on shortly after the patient fell asleep and consisted of jerking of the right side of the face and of the right arm for one to two minutes. She was unable to talk for a few minutes after these attacks.

An electrogram when she was 10 years old showed that the spike focus in the left temporal region was still active.

Comment

The attack patterns, particularly the chewing movements, the ictal and postictal difficulty with speech and the fumbling with clothes, are suggestive of an epileptogenic lesion in the temporal lobe. The right-sided jerking indicated a left-sided focus. The EEG confirmed the presence of a discrete discharging focus in the left temporal region.

The absence of abnormality on clinical examination and the lack of progression made an expanding lesion unlikely. The EEG findings also favored an atrophic lesion. No definite cause was found for the epileptogenic lesion, but the fall at 6 weeks of age may have had some significance in this regard. (It is not uncommon to discover clinical and EEG evidence of an epileptogenic focus without definite indication of any etiological agent.)

EXAMPLE: *Occipital Lesion*
          L.J.L., Clinic No. B-860

This 3 1/2 year old Negro boy was one of fraternal twins and weighed 4 pounds 13 ounces at birth. His neonatal course and development were normal. He was well to 3 5/12 years when his mother noted one afternoon that he suddenly became very still. His head and eyes turned to the left, and when his mother called to him, he said: "I can't see; I can't see." His left arm flexed, his fingers extended and his left lower limb flexed. He then lost consciousness. There was no jerking of his limbs. He remained unconscious for 30 minutes, during which his extremities were limp. On regaining consciousness he complained of headache and was quieter than usual for the remainder of that day. There was no family history of epilepsy.

No abnormality was found on physical examination. Laboratory examinations were normal except for the electroencephalogram. This revealed a discharging slow spike focus in the right occipital region, of the type generally associated with atrophic cortical epileptogenic lesions (fig. 3).

Dilantin was prescribed and no further seizures occurred in a follow-up period of nine months.

Comment

The pattern of attack with impaired vision and turning of the eyes to the opposite side is indicative of a focal right occipital epileptogenic lesion. The electroencephalogram provided supportive evidence of this localization and further indicated the probability of an atrophic lesion.

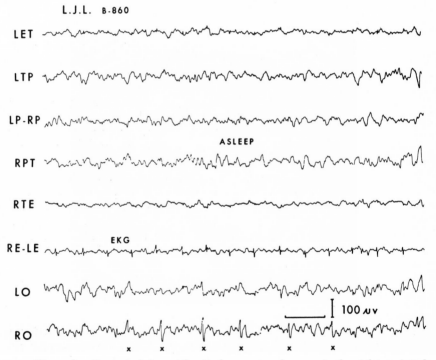

Figure 3.   Repeated slow spike discharges may be seen in the right occipital region (marked by x's). This type of abnormal discharge is usually more evident in sleep recording. Electrocardiographic potentials are present in the RE-LE derivation.

Fig. 4.

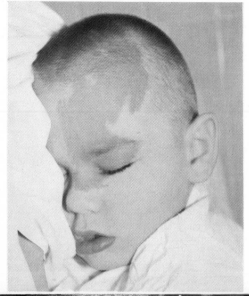

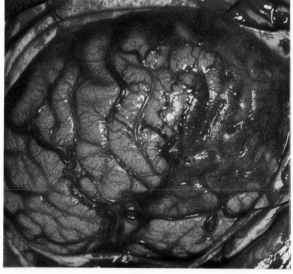

Fig. 5.

Figure 4. The pink birth mark is obvious and outlines the distribution of the first division of the trigeminal nerve.

Figure 5. The red discoloration of the brain in the temporo-parieto-occipital region demonstrates the similarity of the lesion in the brain to that in the skin. The lesion is a malformation of capillaries, encephalotrigeminal angiomatosis.

35

Fig. 6.

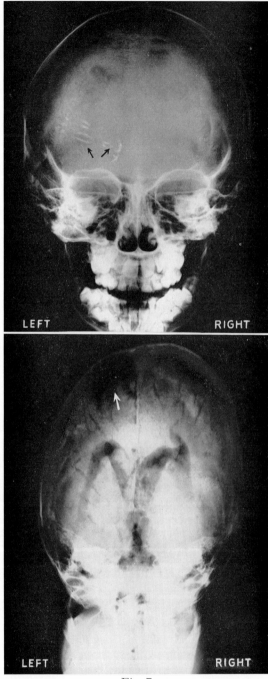

LEFT   RIGHT

LEFT   RIGHT

Fig. 7

Figure 6.   The characteristic "tram line" calcification is evident above the orbit in this film. This is produced by calcification of the malformed cerebral cortex in the occipital region. Note also the smallness of the skull on the side of the lesion, resulting from failure of the underlying brain to grow normally.

Figure 7.   This pneumoencephalogram shows pooling of subarachnoid air over the left occipital pole, which is indicative of atrophy of the cortex beneath it. The smallness of the left cerebral hemisphere is again evident.

This case illustrates the common finding of an atrophic epileptogenic lesion in the absence of any detectable neurological abnormality on examination.

EXAMPLE: *Occipital Lesion*
W.R.B., Clinic No. A-650

From birth this boy had a pink birth mark over his left forehead (fig. 4). At 5 months of age he had his first convulsion; he was afebrile at the time. His eyes turned to the right and there was jerking of his right limbs. Following the seizure he could not move his right side for a few minutes. The attacks recurred and his mother could predict the imminence of a further attack hours before it occurred because the child would appear dazed for periods prior to the seizures. Jerking began in his right foot, spread to the right arm and then to the right side of his face. He screamed immediately after the attacks and he would be "quiet" for several hours afterwards.

There was no family history of seizures but his mother, maternal aunt and maternal grandmother had red birth marks in their occipital regions.

Examination at 7 months showed a hemangioma in the distribution of the first division of the left trigeminal nerve (fig. 4). His right limbs were weak. The first roentgenograms of his skull showed no abnormality. Electroencephalography revealed depression of normal activity in the left parieto-occipital region.

Dilantin and Mebaral were given, but the seizures continued until the patient was 15 months of age. Without medical advice, his parents discontinued the medication at 16 months, and the child remained free of seizures till he was 22 months, when the attacks recurred about once weekly. These consisted of twitching of his right foot for about 15 minutes without loss of consciousness. His mother did not want to give the medication again because she was afraid it would be harmful. In spite of continued attacks, she refused to give medication and also was opposed to surgical intervention.

When the patient was 3 years old his seizures stopped for 10 months, but then recurred. In these attacks his head and eyes first pulled to the right, his right foot turned in and there was a side to side twisting movement of the trunk. At first he had only about one attack daily, but these increased in frequency till he had up to 12 a day.

At 4 years of age the child was extremely hyperactive, could not talk and was not toilet trained.

Dilantin and phenobarbital were prescribed, with a reduction in seizure frequency to about three daily. Other drugs were substituted, including Mebaral, Diamox, Mysoline and Mesantoin but the seizures persisted.

The patient was admitted to the hospital for further investigation at 5 4/12 years.

Repeat roentgenograms of the skull showed calcification in the left occipital region (fig. 6). EEG revealed depression of activity in the left temporo-occipital region, generalized slowing and a right posterior temporal sharp and slow wave focus. Pneumoencephalography showed bilateral ventricular dilatation and a pooling of the air over the left occipital region (fig. 7), indicative of more localized atrophy. Carotid arteriograms were not revealing.

In the hospital the patient was observed to have almost continuous seizures, during which his head turned to the right and jerked for a second or two. He roamed about the room, incessantly crying out. Generalized seizures occurred two to three times daily, in spite of medication.

When he was 5 6/12 years craniotomy was carried out. A malformation of the capillary hemangioma type extended from the occipital lobe to the posterior parietal and temporal regions (fig. 5). Electrocorticography revealed a discharging spike focus in temporal cortex adjacent to the malformation. The malformation and the adjacent abnormally discharging cortex were excised.

Postoperatively there was little change in the hemiparesis and hemianopia, but the patient was much less hyperactive and began to say single words.

Except for a short period postoperatively, he received no anticonvulsants and he has been seizure free for one year, the duration of his follow-up period. He has learned more words and is more aware of his environment. Chlorpromazine was given to curb his hyperactivity. A postoperative EEG showed a left-sided depression of activity but no focal or diffuse epileptiform activity.

Comment

This case demonstrates the effect of "bad brain" on the function of the remaining "normal" tissue, as is indicated by the electroencephalographic findings and by the poorer mental function prior to surgical excision of the lesion.

EXAMPLE: *Frontal Lesion (Tumor)*
        R.J.B., Clinic No B-492

This girl of 3 years was well till she was 14 months, when one day she had twitching of the right side of her face and pulling of her eyes to the right. This lasted only a few seconds and, although the child seemed dazed, she did not lose consciousness. During the next two months the attacks increased in frequency from one a week to one or two a day. Then, in addition to the twitching of the right side of her face and turning of her head and eyes to the right, she would fall and be unable to talk or use her right arm or leg for the duration of the attack and for a short period afterwards.

Phenobarbital was given with a reduction in the frequency of attacks. At 16 to 17 months of age the child began to use her left hand in feeding, whereas before she had used the right hand.

An electroencephalogram at 18 months showed minimal evidence of focal abnormality in the left frontotemporal region. Dilantin was added to the medication. At 2 5/12 years a repeat electrogram showed continuing evidence of a discharging focal abnormality in the left frontotemporal region. When the child was 2 6/12 years the family first noted a dragging of the right leg and weakness of the upper limb.

There was no family history of seizures.

The patient was referred to the Blue Bird Clinic at 3 years, and on examination showed smallness of the right hand and leg. There was a mild right facial weakness and a moderate weakness of her right upper and lower limbs. Myotatic (tendon) reflexes were increased on the right side and there was a right extensor plantar response and sustained ankle clonus. Tone was decreased on the right side. In walking, she had difficulty in lifting her right foot and it slapped the floor when it came down. Sensation was unimpaired to painful stimuli.

A repeat electrogram when she was 3 years showed some slowness and asymmetry between homologous leads, but no further focal or lateralizing signs. Further investigation by angiography and air studies showed evidence of a large mass in the left frontoparietal region. At craniotomy a large cystic tumor was found in the left central region. During surgery the patient had cardiac arrest and died. Autopsy revealed an extensive cystic astrocytoma extending from the frontal to the occipital lobe.

Comment

The seizures were focal in nature and their pattern (twitching of the right side of face and turning of the head and eyes to the right without loss of consciousness) suggested an origin in the left inferior frontal region. This clinical localization was supported by the electrographic evidence of a discharging focus in the left frontotemporal region. The progressive right-sided weakness was suggestive of the possibility of tumor as the etiological agent.

DIFFUSE LESIONS

Diffuse abnormality of the brain may result from such conditions as encephalitis, anoxia, degenerative disease or toxic states. Seizures often are one of the most striking features of the clinical picture. They are likely to occur when the disease process primarily affects the nerve cells, as in the encephalitides or lipoidosis, and are less common when white matter is primarily involved, as in Schilder's disease and other demyelinating processes.

The seizures in diffuse encephalopathies tend to be varied in character. Often a patient will have several types of attacks. He may have at various stages of the disorder, massive spasms and generalized, focal and akinetic seizures. Myoclonus, that is small isolated jerking of muscle groups, is also a common feature in such patients.

Of all laboratory studies, electroencephalography is the most productive in such cases. The character of the findings varies with the stage of the disease process at the time of the study. Initially, the record may show a high voltage generalized slow pattern with paroxysmal slow bursts. Later, generalized spike and slow wave patterns of various types may develop. Roentgenology seldom provides much diagnostic information in cases of this kind.

EXAMPLE: *Diffuse Lesion*
W.R.R., Clinic No. B-740

This boy was almost 7 years of age when his vision began to deteriorate. Mental deterioration appeared soon after the visual difficulty was noted, and this too was gradually progressive. He became weak, stumbled and lost his balance easily.

At 9 years of age he began to have convulsions. In these attacks he would call to his mother and then his head turned to the left; he became rigid, with his eyes rolled up, and fell in a generalized clonic convulsion lasting about one minute. He then slept for 30 to 60 minutes and on arousing was disoriented. He had these attacks about every six weeks. Mesantoin and phenobarbital reduced the frequency of his attacks.

He had two younger siblings with a similar history of an onset of blindness at 7 years, convulsions at 9 years and progressive mental deterioration.

Examination at 14 years of age showed the boy to have the mental ability of a child of 5. His speech was slurred. He could perceive light but not hand movements. The optic discs were pale. Both retinae were pale with peripheral, reticulate deposits of black pigment. The retinal vessels were very thin.

His pupils were dilated, were equal and reacted sluggishly to light. A fixation type of fine nystagmus was present at rest. His power and coordination were unimpaired, and tone was slightly increased in his upper limbs. The myotatic reflexes were increased bilaterally, with bilateral nonsustained ankle clonus; both plantar responses were flexor. No abnormality of sensation was detected. He had a wide-based, slightly stiff and hesitant gait.

Slight generalized dilatation of the lateral ventricles was demonstrated on pneumoencephalography. The spinal fluid contained 6 polys and 4 lymphocytes per cubic millimeter and the protein content was 64 mg. per cent.

Electroencephalography revealed a continuous generalized slow dysrhythmia with recurrent paroxysmal frontal dominant bursts of high voltage 2 per second waves, and occasional slow spike and wave complexes.

Mesantoin and phenobarbital were continued. The patient had generalized seizures about every second month and occasional brief myoclonic jerks. Two repeat EEG studies when he was 15 5/12 and 16 4/12 years showed essentially no change.

Comment

The patient showed the characteristic findings of lipoidosis of the Spielmeyer-Vogt type, including the familial incidence, the seizures and the gradual progression of visual and mental deterioration. The electroencephalogram was in keeping with a diffuse process.

The seizures were much less incapacitating than the blindness, the mental deterioration and the clumsiness.

EXAMPLE: *Diffuse Lesion*
> P. J. H., Clinic No. B-402

This girl was well until she was 5 1/12 years, when she began to awaken at night crying. A few days later she was noted to stumble frequently, to fall and to be unsteady in the use of her hands. A few days later the child became confused and fearful and her speech was slurred. She was alternately drowsy and restless.

There were frequent scattered jerking movements of her limbs and face during sleep. When awake, her eyelids would suddenly droop and she would drop almost to the ground before catching herself. She then began to have episodes in which she suddenly fell backward. Vomiting occurred occasionally and she became incontinent.

After about a month the symptoms appeared to clear a little. She was admitted to a hospital where she was found to be hyperactive and slightly unsteady in her gait. She had bilateral papilledema. Her arm movements were incoordinate. She had an electroencephalogram at 5 2/12 years which showed a paroxysmal generalized dysrhythmia of a fast and slow type and shifting foci of sharp wave activity in sleep. A right carotid angiogram and a ventriculogram were carried out and showed no definite evidence of abnormality, although the ventricles appeared small.

She was transferred to the Blue Bird Clinic for further study. She was confused and fearful and her speech was slurred. Fundoscopic examination showed bilateral papilledema. Her motor power was reduced generally with no particular focal weakness. The myotatic reflexes were slightly increased, the left knee jerk was slightly more active than the right and there was bilateral unsustained ankle clonus. Sensation was thought to be intact for pain, touch and vibration. Position sense and two-point discrimination were not tested because of poor cooperation. The patient walked unsteadily, veered to one side or the other or fell forwards. At times she appeared to jerk backwards suddenly. Periodically her eyelids would momentarily droop and she became limp.

A repeat EEG showed more prolonged and slower paroxysmal generalized bursts with almost continuous very slow frontal activity (fig. 8). Several lumbar punctures were performed, some showing increased pressure and cell count. A paretic gold curve (5554321000) was present. Another EEG at 5 3/12 years was more abnormal than the preceding one, with more frequent generalized high voltage paroxysmal bursts.

The patient was discharged on Dilantin and phenobarbital, and she continued to deteriorate. She was unable to state her wants and did not use her right side as much as her left. Generalized convulsions occurred, as well as isolated jerking movements of her limbs.

When seen at 5 4/12 years, she had practically continuous attacks of sudden abduction of her arms with flexion of her knees and thighs. She also had episodic

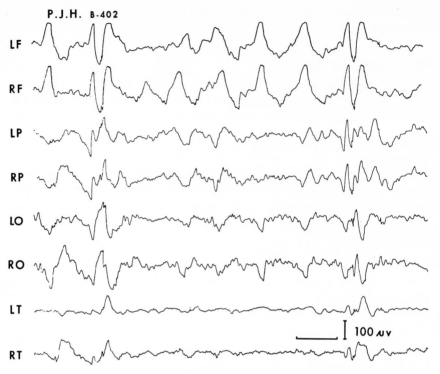

Figure 8. This electroencephalogram shows almost continuous high voltage slow waves of irregular and often sharp configuration in the frontal leads, and recurrent sharp and slow wave discharges maximal in the frontal region but reflected in all leads. This type of electroencephalogram is considered indicative of a diffuse degenerative process.

turning of her head to the right, blinking or sudden loss of postural tone. She kept her right fingers flexed. A grasp reflex was present in the right hand. Tone was increased in the right limbs and the right biceps jerk was brisker than the left. The plantar responses were flexor. Both optic discs had indistinct edges and the retinal veins were full. A repeat EEG showed less bifrontal slow activity. She became bedridden, had intermittent convulsions and gradually deteriorated to her death at 5 8/12 years.

A postmortem examination of her brain showed subacute inclusion body encephalitis.

Comment

The great variety of seizure patterns and the scattered myoclonic and akinetic attacks in particular favored a diffuse process as the basis of the epilepsy. The mental deterioration and the character of the electrographic abnormality supported the diagnosis of diffuse and severe cerebral disease.

It is of interest that the EEG helped to rule out a diagnosis of brain tumor early in the disease.

MULTIPLE FOCAL LESIONS

If a patient has attacks which have differing aura and attack patterns, possibly with different sides of the body being involved in different attacks, it is probable that more than one site of origin of epileptic discharge is present. A large tumor may have multiple zones of epileptogenic activity around its periphery, but the most common situation in which multifocal epilepsy occurs in children is as a residual of a diffuse encephalopathy resulting from infection, anoxia, toxin and trauma. After recovery from the acute stages of a diffuse encephalopathy, some focal regions of the cortex may develop a localized hyperirritable state which gives rise to spontaneous seizure discharge.

EXAMPLE: *Multiple Focal Lesions*
R.P., Clinic No. B-338

This boy of 6 years was perfectly well till he was 2 years of age, when he vomited for two days and then began to have convulsions. In these seizures his eyes turned up, his left shoulder drooped and his left leg dragged. He then lost consciousness and there were clonic movements beginning in his left arm and leg, later becoming generalized. He was admitted to a hospital in a comatose state and received oxygen for two days. On discharge three months later, he no longer talked and had occasional convulsions. At 3 years of age, he had a severe convulsion and was again admitted to hospital where he was noted to have mental retardation and a lead line in his gums. It was found that at 1 year of age he had begun eating the paint from the woodwork both inside and outside the home. There was no family history of seizures. Roentgenograms of the long bones showed lead lines, and determinations of lead in the blood, spinal fluid, urine and bone showed significant amounts to be present.

An electroencephalogram at 2 8/12 years showed no abnormality. A repeat study at 3 5/12 years revealed diffuse slowing and multiple foci of low voltage spike activity. At 6 10/12 years an EEG showed a single active left occipital spike focus.

Physical examination at 6 10/12 years revealed mental retardation and great distractibility. He was given Dilantin and phenobarbital with reduction in the number of attacks. In the attacks the child would run to his mother saying that he was sick; his head and eyes turned to the left, and he became apneic and then blue. He had other attacks in which he became pale, asked for water and then lay down. He was sleepy after these attacks. At 7 5/12 years a repeat EEG showed the same left occipital spike focus.

At 7 10/12 years he began having right-sided seizures, with jerking movements beginning in the right hand. His medication was changed to Dilantin, Mesantoin and Mebaral without much improvement. At 8 years he still had attacks consisting of epigastric and respiratory distress, pallor, brief unconsciousness and sometimes stiffness or slight jerking. The seizures continued, with the warning of a right-sided headache, turning of head to the right and flexion of the right forearm. The patient lost consciousness and might remain unconscious for five minutes. After the attacks he was weak and limp and often slept. For 15 to 30 minutes after the attacks he complained of abdominal pain. Medication was changed to Mysoline, Diamox, Mebaral and Mesantoin with lessened severity of the attacks.

EEG at 8 8/12 years revealed independent discharging spike foci in the left occipital and left inferior temporal regions.

At 9 years the patient's I.Q. was 42. Attacks continued about twice weekly with aura of headache followed by a turning of his head to the right and flexion of the right forearm. With the onset of the movements there was loss of consciousness. Postictally he was weak and limp and complained of abdominal pain.

At 10 years of age Celontin was started, with temporary improvement in his seizures.

Comment

The varying pattern of this patient's seizures indicated multiple epileptogenic lesions. Some of the electroencephalograms showed the presence of multiple epileptogenic foci. Multifocal epilepsy is commonly the result of remote severe brain damage, which in this case was due to acute lead intoxication. The mental retardation was a result of the neuronal loss in the acute phase of the encephalopathy.

REFERENCES

1. Fender, F. A.: Anoxia and the convulsive state. California Med., 71:103, 1949.
2. Smith, B., Robinson, G. C. and Lennox, W. G.: Acquired epilepsy. A study of 535 cases. Neurology, 4:19, 1954.
3. Chao, D. D.: Seizures in infancy and early childhood. M. Clin. North America, 42:399, 1958.
4. Druckman, R., Chao, D. D., Kellaway, P.: Transient epileptogenic encephalopathy. M. Clin. North America, 42:455, 1958.
5. Scott, J. S. and Kellaway, P.: Epilepsy of focal origin in childhood. M. Clin. North America, 42:415, 1958.

CHAPTER 6

Massive Spasms

THE TERM *massive spasm* refers to a type of seizure characterized by a sudden and usually strong contraction of most of the body musculature. The seizure may be momentary in duration, but more often each spasm lasts a second or more. The usual pattern is flexion and adduction of the limbs and a doubling up of the body. These have been called "jackknife" attacks. Extensor spasms occur less often, with extension of the neck and limbs and often abduction of the upper limbs. This type of attack resembles an exaggerated Moro reflex. There may be a mixture of extensor and flexor movements, a "mixed" massive spasm.

These seizures are fairly common in the first two years of life, occurring less frequently than generalized convulsions but about as often as focal seizures. The age of onset is usually between 1 and 6 months, but these attacks may come on up to the age of 2 years and rarely later than this. The attacks may consist of a series of spasms or occur singly. Attacks occurring in series generally begin with strong and prolonged contractions which become successively less strong and more widely spaced until they stop. A cry commonly accompanies the more severe massive spasms. Pupillary dilatation, nystagmus, sweating, pallor, flushing, cyanosis and an appearance of fear, grimacing or laughter may occur in these seizures. The fre-

45

quency varies from one attack in several days to 200 or more attacks daily.

Various factors tend to precipitate this type of seizure. The commonest of these is the twilight state between sleep and wakefulness. Infection and fever, sudden noise, excitement, handling, feeding and excessive heat also may bring on these attacks.

When the attacks are frequent, the patients are often hyperirritable and continuously fretful. Sometimes in these periods, the patients assume rigid postures with stiffly outstretched limbs which may tremble. They may become opisthotonic and remain in this state for hours or even days. Medication lessening the severity and frequency of the massive spasms will also reduce or abolish the opisthotonus and hyperirritability.

Other types of seizure may precede, accompany or follow the massive spasms. The massive spasms also change in pattern and frequency with time. The usual change is from the flexor to mixed and extensor types. The massive spasms may persist for weeks and then spontaneously cease. The attacks may stop, only to reappear a few weeks or months later. The first sign of improvement is a reduction in the number of serial attacks; even the isolated spasms will eventually occur less frequently and only in response to some external stimulus, such as a sudden noise.

Massive spasms usually disappear by 3 years of age, but attacks of this type have been known to persist up to the age of 8 years. The attacks are more likely to persist where the brain damage is so great that development is arrested. Seizures of other types may follow the cessation of massive spasms and are most frequently focal motor in type, although generalized attacks are also common.

Patients with massive spasms generally show some degree of motor and mental retardation. Frequently, the parents bring the infant to the physician because of slowness of development rather than because of the attacks, which they dismiss as colic or other benign features of infant life. The degree of motor and mental retardation appears to be proportional to the severity and frequency of the seizures. The onset of spasms may mark a regression in the development of the infant, and a cessation of attacks will often be followed by an improvement in his physical and mental development. Even with complete cessation of seizures, however, it is very unusual for mentality to reach full development. The majority of patients have signs of cerebral injury, but these may not be obvious in early life. Hemiplegia, spasticity and athetosis are found in a large proportion of these patients. Hypotonia, nystagmus and microcephaly are also relatively frequent findings.

The electroencephalogram usually shows a pathognomonic pattern known as hypsarhythmia. This is characterized by a diffusely abnormal pattern without periods of normal activity, with bursts of irregular generalized high voltage slow and sharp activity, which are often immediately followed by a short period of relative electrographic silence, by shifting foci of polyspike discharge and by poor interhemispheric synchrony and symmetry. When the high voltage slow bursts show good synchrony and when some normal activity is present in the waking records, the pattern is called modified hypsarhythmia. Less frequently, other electrographic abnormalities may occur in massive spasms, particularly generalized slow spike wave variants. Rarely, the electroencephalogram may be normal early in the course of massive spasms. The EEG may revert to normal in time.

Pneumoencephalography commonly reveals evidence of cerebral atrophy. Other laboratory investigations do not show pertinent abnormality.

Rarely, a patient with massive spasms may show remarkable recovery after the spasms stop and may develop normally. The possibility of a benign outcome is greater with the less severe, prolonged and frequent attacks and the later onset of the seizures. An electroencephalogram which shows some periods of relatively normal activity is also encouraging.

Massive spasms appear to be a manifestation of brain damage sustained early in life, which is usually diffuse and severe. The causes of brain damage are of several types and may operate in prenatal, natal or early postnatal life. They include bleeding or infection in utero and congenital malformations. At birth, anoxia and trauma are common etiological agents, while in postnatal life, trauma, encephalitis and encephalopathy secondary to systemic infection and dehydration are frequent causes of this syndrome. The cause of the brain injury is often unknown. Indeed, the nature of the injury may never be established; this is true in about 30 per cent of patients with massive spasms.

Treatment of these patients is generally very difficult, since the spasms are usually quite resistant to therapy. In our hands, a combination of Gemonil and Mebaral has been the most effective treatment. Meprobamate and Celontin have also occasionally proved effective. The dosages are given in the Drug Table, page 138.

EXAMPLE: *Massive Spasms*
R.H., Clinic No. B-380

This boy was delivered at term. The placenta was small and green; the umbilical cord was also small (the thickness of a pencil) and olive green. Resuscitation was difficult and the neonate was placed in the incubator and given oxygen. When brought to his mother for a feeding, he stopped breathing and became cyanotic. Two similar spells occurred in the next three days.

In the first three months of life, the patient had twitching movements of his right leg. At 12 months he had frequent episodes in which his head suddenly dropped forward. The head nodding continued, and at 14 months he had attacks in which his face appeared masklike and he was unresponsive for several seconds. At 15 months his head nodding and face stiffening were accompanied by a stiffening and throwing forward of the upper limbs, as well as a loss of consciousness. These attacks would last from 3 to 60 seconds and occurred frequently throughout the day, particularly upon awakening. Phenobarbital was given, which reduced the number of attacks.

The child rolled over at 12 months, sat alone and crawled at 14 months and walked at 16 months.

On examination at 17 months, the fontanels were closed and his head circumference was small (43.8 cm.). His movements were incoordinate, he walked unsteadily, and was considered retarded. An electroencephalogram at that time showed the continuously epileptiform, diffusely abnormal pattern known as hypsarhythmia (fig. 9).

Tridione and Mebaral were given, but the Tridione was discontinued because of granulocytopenia and a lack of effectiveness. The patient continued to have attacks of stiffening of his neck, head nodding or jackknifing of his whole body. Mysoline was added to the Mebaral but the attacks continued at a frequency of about 20 daily. Milontin and Mebaral were then tried with little effect.

At 2 3/12 years, the child still had flexor and extensor massive spasms and he began to have other seizures in which his left arm and leg jerked and he cried out. After these episodes he seemed exhausted. Mebaral and Gemonil were given, and there was a decrease in the frequency of attacks. When he was awake, the attacks consisted of a twisting of his mouth, rolling up of his eyes with a flicker-

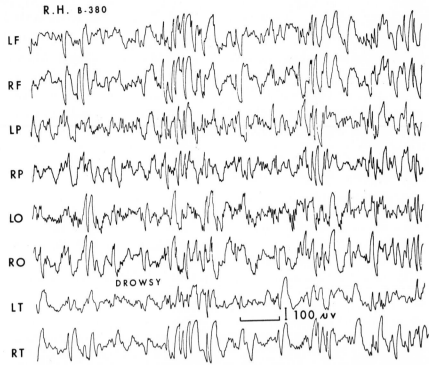

Figure 9. This sample shows the generalized high voltage slow, sharp and spike activity which characterizes hypsarhythmia. Note also the lack of symmetry in the activity of homologous regions, which is especially marked in the temporal regions.

ing of the eyelids, flexion of his arms and legs and a jackknifing of his body. During sleep, there was only mild flexion of his arms and legs.

With the decrease in the frequency of seizures, the child showed an improved motor and mental ability. At 2 5/12 years he could hold a fork, throw a ball and go upstairs.

Seizures stopped for two and one-half months, but recurred. The patient then had momentary extension of the neck and about two brief head-nodding attacks daily. He also had episodes in which he slowly fell to the floor.

The EEG at 2 11/12 years was essentially unchanged. Diamox was added to the Mebaral and Gemonil, and shortly afterward, at 3 years of age, the child's seizures ceased. He continued to be moderately retarded mentally and quite hyperactive.

After five months without a seizure, the mother stopped the medication. Meprobamate was given for hyperactivity, but had no effect. His EEG at 4 years showed a generalized high voltage random spike and wave pattern, with higher voltage on the right. There were episodes of rhythmic 2½ per second spike and wave activity showing right-sided predominance and occasional right frontal random spikes.

When the child was 4 6/12 years seizures recurred. These involved a stiffening of the arms and legs followed by giggling. Each seizure lasted for one-half to one minute and he had two attacks daily. Seizures increased to six to eight daily, and began with giggling which increased in intensity. The upper limbs then extended and his knees adducted. He lost consciousness but did not usually fall during the attacks. After these seizures he was quiet for a few minutes. He continued to be hyperactive and had frequent temper tantrums. When he was 4 7/12 years his head circumference was 48 cm., he was clumsy and could not speak. Chlorpromazine was prescribed for the hyperactivity and Celontin for the seizures, with moderate improvement.

Comment

The wide range of seizure patterns, which included focal motor, head-nodding, massive spasm and giggling attacks, the severe mental retardation, the hyperactivity and the electroencephalographic findings of hypsarhythmia and variant, slow spike and wave abnormality, indicated widespread and severe brain damage. The presumptive cause of the brain damage was anoxia in utero secondary to the hypoplastic placenta.

The difficulty encountered in control of the seizures is common in this type of patient.

REFERENCES

1. West, W. J.: On a peculiar form of infantile convulsion. Lancet, 1:724, 1841.
2. Gibbs, E. L., Fleming, M. M. and Gibbs, F. A.: Diagnosis and prognosis of hypsarhythmia and infantile spasms. Pediatrics, 13:66, 1954.
3. Druckman, R. and Chao, D.: Massive spasms in infancy and childhood. Epilepsia, 4:61, 1955.
4. Chao, D. D., Taylor, F. M. and Druckman, R.: Massive spasms. J. Pediat., 50:670, 1957.
5. Baird, H. W. and Borofsky, L. G.: Infantile myoclonic seizures. J. Pediat., 50:332, 1957.

CHAPTER 7

Idiopathic (Genetic) Epilepsy

IDIOPATHIC epilepsy is a condition which is characterized by specific seizure types, definite age incidence, lack of abnormal neurological findings, characteristic electroencephalographic pattern and a familial incidence. To these criteria may be added one which can seldom be tested, namely the absence of anatomical abnormality of the brain at autopsy.

Other terms which have been used for this group include cryptogenic, genetic and centrencephalic or central. The term *idiopathic* means "springing from itself"; this is apt in that it emphasizes the essential feature of this type, the lack of any demonstrable lesion of the brain. The term *genetic* emphasizes the importance of hereditary factors, but it has connotations which are pragmatically undesirable. *Cryptogenic* merely means of unknown origin, but while one may not be able to define the cause in a particular case, the evidence from the pattern of the seizures or from laboratory studies may clearly indicate an underlying cerebral lesion. Thus, not all cryptogenic epilepsy is idiopathic epilepsy.

The term *centrencephalic* or *central* refers to the probable localization or site of origin of the epileptic discharge in the center of the brain (thalamic intralaminar system), but it does not define the

51

causative factor. This term is too inclusive for equation with idio-pathic epilepsy, for while it is true that the epileptic discharge in idiopathic epilepsy probably has its origin in the diencephalon, this term would also include seizures due to organic factors, such as lesions in the thalamus or in the region of the third ventricle.

The various types of seizures which occur in idiopathic epilepsy are described in the following pages.

Absence or Lapse Attacks

The patients in the idiopathic group with only momentary lapses of consciousness constitute the purest culture of idiopathic epilepsy. Generally, the onset of attacks occurs between 4 and 10 years of age. These lapses may be very frequent, occurring up to hundreds of times daily. Their frequency led earlier neurologists to refer to them as pyknolepsy ("pyknos" means frequent). The duration of each seizure is rarely more than three to five seconds, but longer attacks do occasionally occur. Rarely, these attacks may occur in such close succession and for such prolonged periods that consciousness may be continuously impaired, the patient remaining in a continuously clouded and confused state. This is the so-called serial petit mal or petit mal status.

Patients with pure absence attacks generally show no abnormal physical findings and are mentally normal. These patients have the best prognosis, with the seizures usually decreasing in their teens and disappearing completely before their twenties.

Patients with lapse attacks may also have generalized seizures. In this group the lapse attacks commonly decrease as the child grows older, but the generalized seizures may continue after the lapses have ceased.

The electroencephalographic abnormality in patients with lapse attacks is striking and characteristic. Bursts of generalized bilaterally synchronous 3 per second spike and wave complexes appear, usually against a background of normal activity. The frequency may be 4 per second at the onset of a burst and slow to 2 per second at its termination. The slow component is more constant than the spike, and paroxysmal bursts of generalized rhythmic 3 per cent activity may predominate. Short paroxysmal bursts of such activity may produce no obvious clinical manifestation, but recent evidence indicates that subtle changes in mental efficiency occur during these episodes. Clinical attacks are usually not evident unless the bursts are of a duration of three or more seconds.

Skull films and pneumoencephalograms are characteristically normal, and indications for the latter are extremely rare in this group.

Factors precipitating this type of clinical and electrographic attack include hyperventilation, strong or flickering lights, hypoglycemia and emotional excitement. In this connection it may be noted that exercise involving overbreathing may bring on attacks. Attentiveness tends to inhibit these attacks.

EXAMPLE: *Lapse Attacks*
        D.R.N., Clinic No. B-320

At 3 years of age, this boy began to have attacks in which he abruptly stopped whatever he was doing, his eyes stared straight ahead or rolled up and his eyelids blinked slowly. He was unresponsive during these episodes, which lasted several seconds and occurred one to five times daily. Later he began to urinate with each attack. The seizures were precipitated by excitement, fear, pleasure or pain.

At 9 months of age, the patient had had a short generalized tonic-clonic convulsion during a febrile illness.

The boy's maternal aunt had "blank" spells with an onset at 4 to 5 years of age, and at 14 years she had generalized seizures and several bouts of status epilepticus. Another maternal aunt had generalized seizures beginning at 16 years, and a maternal great aunt also had generalized seizures.

On examination at 12 years of age, the boy was intelligent and showed no neurological abnormality. He was observed in two of his attacks. In these he stopped his gum-chewing and stared straight ahead for several seconds, his eyelids blinking rhythmically. After he recovered, he did not recall anything that had been said to him during this period. His electroencephalogram showed paroxysmal generalized 3 per second spike and wave dysrhythmia (fig. 10).

Tridione, 300 mg. three times daily, was prescribed with a decrease in seizure frequency to two a day. The dose of Tridione was increased to 300 mg. four times daily and no further seizure occurred in the next two years. Medication was then discontinued and the patient remained free of seizures over the next five months, the duration of his follow-up.

An EEG at 14 4/12 years showed an occipital dominant slow dysrhythmia without evidence of spike and wave activity. A further EEG at 15 7/12 years was considered to be normal.

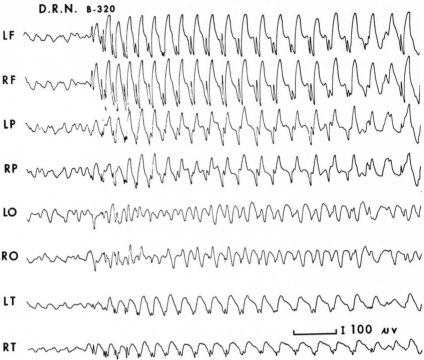

Figure 10. This electroencephalographic sample shows a sudden burst out of a normal background of generalized but frontal dominant, spike and slow wave discharge. Note that the paroxysmal spike and slow wave activity slows from an initial frequency of about 4 per second to approximately 2 1/2 per second at the end of the burst.

Comment

This boy's seizures were typical of the lapse attacks of idiopathic epilepsy in the age of onset, in the staring with associated blinking and in the family history of seizures. The electroencephalogram showed the pattern characteristic of this type of epilepsy, the paroxysmal generalized 3 per second spike and wave dysrhythmia. The only unusual feature of his attacks was the incontinence, which rarely accompanies this type of attack. As is the general rule in patients of this group, a good response to Tridione was obtained.

Myoclonic Attacks

Momentary jerks of limbs or even of individual groups of muscles may occur in patients with idiopathic epilepsy. These may happen without apparent impairment of consciousness or with a typical absence. The eye blinking which often accompanies absence attacks is probably a similar phenomenon. Myoclonic jerks tend to occur more frequently in the morning and on going to sleep. In patients with both generalized and myoclonic attacks, the myoclonic jerks often occur in series preceding a generalized seizure, and may serve as a warning of the impending convulsion. Normal individuals may have occasional myoclonic jerks in drowsiness or light sleep.

The electroencephalogram in this condition characteristically shows bursts of generalized multiple spike and 3 per second slow wave complexes.

Myoclonic jerks without associated lapse attacks are more common in symptomatic than in idiopathic epilepsy. When myoclonic jerks constitute the predominant seizure pattern, the diagnosis of some degenerative cerebral disorder should be considered.

EXAMPLE: *Lapse and Myoclonic Attacks*
I.R., Clinic No. B-373

This boy was 4 5/12 years of age when his mother noted that he was having brief "blank" spells. At first these occurred about twice daily but their frequency gradually increased. In the attacks the boy stopped whatever he was doing, blinked his eyes and nodded his head once or twice. If he was being held at the time of the attack, a very slight rhythmic jerking of the muscles of his upper limbs could be felt, but there was no grossly visible movement of these extremities. An EEG at 4 11/12 years revealed a paroxysmal generalized 3 per second spike and wave and multiple spike and wave dysrhythmia. His pediatrician prescribed Mebaral and Tridione and the frequency of attacks was reduced, but 12 days later he developed a drug rash and these medications were stopped. Mebaral and Dilantin were given, but again a rash developed and medication was discontinued. Paradione produced a rash, fever and vomiting. Mebaral alone was given but there was no improvement. Milontin and Tridione were then prescribed but discontinued 10 days later when the child developed a generalized rash, fever and vomiting. Mysoline was tried next without improvement in seizures, but with the production of a rash and fever. Electroencephalography at 5 6/12 years showed much more frequent bursts of spike and wave activity and little activity of normal character. Medication was completely discontinued, and the boy started to have 10 or more seizures hourly.

The child's birth and development were normal. There was no family history of epilepsy or other neurological disorder.

Examination in the Blue Bird Clinic at 5 7/12 years showed no abnormal findings except for frequent seizures, characterized by head nodding, eye blinking and loss of consciousness for about three seconds. The patient was admitted to the hospital where he continued to have seizures every few minutes. Ammonium chloride and Dexedrine were given without effect. These were stopped and the ketogenic diet started. His seizures decreased to a frequency of one to three a day. A further EEG showed slight improvement with shorter bursts of paroxysmal generalized 3 per second spike and slow wave abnormality.

The boy was discharged from the hospital, and the adequacy of the ketogenic diet was checked by the mother who tested the urine daily for ketonuria. Seizure frequency was reduced to one or two daily, and the attacks finally stopped completely when he was 6 years of age. At 7 4/12 years the proportion of fats to other foodstuffs was reduced from 4 to 1 (by weight) to 3 to 1. The child continued free of seizures and his diet was liberalized gradually so that at 8 6/12 years he was taking a normal diet. He remained free of seizures for the next six months, the duration of his follow-up period. An EEG at 8 10/12 years showed several episodes of 14 and 6 per second positive spike activity during sleep, but no other abnormality.

Comment

Although there was some improvement in the lapse attacks with the use of Tridione, the idiosyncrasy to this and other drugs made it necessary to resort to the ketogenic diet before control of his seizures was attained. This case demonstrates the effectiveness of the diet when rigidly carried out in selected cases.

Akinetic Attacks

Akinetic attacks are seizures characterized by sudden, brief loss of postural tone. The patient may merely slump a little before catching himself or he may be to his knees or on the ground before tone returns. Consciousness is probably lost momentarily in these attacks, but this is a difficult point to determine. In its simplest form there may be only a sudden nodding of the head. This type of seizure should be clearly differentiated from the type in which the patient becomes limp and gradually sinks to the floor, remaining unconscious for seconds or even minutes. These syncopal-like attacks have an entirely different significance (p. 60).

Although akinetic attacks may occur in idiopathic epilepsy, our experience indicates that this seizure pattern is more commonly associated with symptomatic epilepsy and occurs most often in severe diffuse encephalopathies.

Generalized Seizures

Generalized seizures may occur alone or in association with lapse, myoclonic or akinetic attacks. They show a much lesser tendency to spontaneous remission in later life than do these other types of seizures.

To qualify with certainty as idiopathic epilepsy, generalized seizures should have no localizing or lateralizing features. The existence of any type of aura should immediately suggest that the patient has symptomatic epilepsy, until proved otherwise, although it is possible that an epigastric aura such as a rising sensation, fullness or vague discomfort may occur in idiopathic epilepsy. Occasionally there may be a prodrome of headache or irritability. If the seizure is not a prolonged one, there should be no evidence of localized weakness following an attack, although in the immediate postictal period there may be some transient abnormal neurological findings, such as an abnormal plantar response. As is the rule in idiopathic epilepsy, patients are mentally and neurologically normal.

The electroencephalogram in these patients may show generalized 3 per second multiple spike and wave bursts or paroxysmal polyspike bursts without slow activity, but there is no electrographic pattern with which it is specifically correlated. Indeed, many patients with idiopathic epilepsy who have only generalized seizures show normal interseizure electroencephalograms (8–10 per cent).

REFERENCES

1. Adie, W. J.: Pyknolepsy: a form of epilepsy occurring in children with a good prognosis. Brain, 47:96, 1924.
2. Lennox, W. G.: Sixty-six twin pairs affected by seizures. A. Research Nerv. and Ment. Dis., Proc., 26:11, 1947.
3. Penfield, W. and Jasper, H.: Highest level seizures. A. Research Nerv. and Ment. Dis., Proc., 26:252, 1947.
4. Shimazono, Y., Hirai, T., Okuma, T., Fukuda, T. and Yamamasu, E.: Disturbances of consciousness in petit mal epilepsy. Epilepsia, 2:49,1953.
5. Lennox, W. G. and Jolly, D. H.: Seizures, brain waves and intelligence tests of epileptic twins. Assoc. Res. Nerv. Ment. Dis., 33:325, 1954.
6. Kellaway, P. and Druckman, R.: Idiopathic epilepsy: criteria for diagnosis. M. Clin. North America, 42:375, 1958.

CHAPTER 8

Convulsive Equivalent
Attacks

CLASSICALLY, epilepsy has been considered a disorder characterized by attacks involving convulsive movements or loss of consciousness, or both. It is now established that a wide variety of symptoms,
which are quite unlike a convulsion and which do not involve
changes in consciousness, may have their origin in paroxysmal disturbances in the brain akin to those which underlie a convulsive
seizure. These attacks, which may be as simple as a headache, are
called "convulsive equivalents" because of the similarity of the underlying mechanism in the brain to convulsive disorder. The term "epileptic equivalent" is a misnomer, because the attacks are not
equivalent to epilepsy but are equivalent to the convulsion; they are
epileptic in that they have their origin in a spontaneous massive
ganglionic discharge in the brain which differs from that of the
classic epileptic seizure only in terms of localization and spread.

This relationship was recognized quite early solely on clinical
grounds, but because the symptoms differed so greatly from the
usual concept of an epileptic seizure, they were classified as belong-
ing in the "borderlands of epilepsy." The advent of electroenceph-

alography provided objective evidence that these clinical insights were correct and that a wide variety of symptoms, often of a purely subjective nature, were caused by the same type of neuronal storm in the brain as that underlying a convulsion.

Paroxysmal attacks of abdominal pain have been the most widely accepted form of convulsive equivalent and have been designated as "abdominal epilepsy." It is probable, however, that headache occurs more commonly as a convulsive equivalent. Both are much more common in children than in adults. Usually the headache or abdominal pain is only a part of a total pattern and the patient more often has accompanying autonomic disturbances, including pallor or flushing, elevation or depression of temperature, vomiting, pupillary changes, sweating, increased peristalsis, increased thirst or hunger, salivation and incontinence. Limpness, or, less often, generalized weakness, may be a feature of the attacks. The autonomic and pain features of the attacks may be accompanied by changes in mood and occasionally of behavior, with the development in rare instances of sudden aggressive and destructive episodes and even of rage attacks.

It is not uncommon to find patients, especially children, who have attacks in which nearly all the autonomic features are present. Full-blown attacks may consist of headache, eye pain, abdominal pain, vomiting, pallor, weakness or limpness, dizziness, temperature variations and behavior changes followed by sleepiness. The sleep which follows an attack is often abnormally deep and prolonged. The more general pattern is for the patient to have only the pain and perhaps one or two of the autonomic features in most of his attacks. On the other hand, patients in this group may experience attacks of unconsciousness or even a generalized seizure. The episodes of unconsciousness may occur at the height of the autonomic and pain attack or as an isolated event. The same is true of the generalized seizures. In practice it is often the advent of such an attack which points to the real nature of the paroxysmal episodes of pain and autonomic disturbance.

Precipitating factors are overventilation, brought on by such things as exercise or crying, and sleep. Emotional upset and blows to the head also appear to be effective agents in bringing on attacks. The fact that emotional upsets or minor head injuries can precipitate these attacks should be stressed, because the presence of this type of initial feature may confuse the diagnostic picture.

Characteristically, the physical examination reveals no evidence of abnormality. Laboratory studies other than electroencephalography are normal. The EEG often provides the only objective evidence to support the diagnosis, but a single negative study should not be considered to rule out a convulsive equivalent disorder, because the abnormalities associated with this clinical syndrome may not be easy to demonstrate and it may be necessary to do more than one study, including sleep, in order to demonstrate clearly defined electrographic abnormality. Occasionally, it may even be necessary to resort to recording at the time of an attack in order to prove the diagnosis.

The significant electroencephalographic abnormalities are: (1) 14 and 6 per second positive spikes, and (2) spontaneous paroxysmal slow activity and a marked and excessively prolonged reaction to overbreathing. These EEG findings are usually present between seizures. During the attacks the electroencephalogram reveals much more abnormality, either almost continuous generalized high voltage slow activity or more frequent episodes of 14 and 6 per second positive spike discharge. Other types of EEG abnormality are sometimes found, such as discharging spike foci, but as yet there is insufficient evidence to indicate any direct causal relation of focal cortical abnormality to the autonomic attacks.

Depending upon the localization of pain and the nature of the autonomic disturbance, the differential diagnosis may include acute abdominal conditions, such as intussusception where abdominal pain and vomiting are prominent, or intracranial expanding lesions where headache and stupor are presenting features. Episodic behavioral disorder may be confused with purely psychogenic disturbance. The recurrent paroxysmal character of the attacks, followed by sleep, favors the diagnosis of convulsive equivalent disorder. Roentgenological study of the gastrointestinal and urinary systems may be necessary in order to rule out local pathology. Similarly, skull roentgenograms and even air encephalography may rarely be required to eliminate the possibility of a space-occupying intracranial lesion.

Disturbed function at a diencephalic level is believed to provide the basic mechanism of this clinical syndrome. This localization is based on the nature of the symptoms (autonomic), which have a prominent hypothalamic character, on the type of electrographic abnormality, which is believed to originate in the diencephalon, and on occasional autopsy findings of abnormality involving the diencephalon.

There are many possible causes of this syndrome. Any etiological agent capable of disturbing function in the hypothalamic-thalamic region can produce convulsive equivalent disorder. Post-traumatic sequelae and developmental anomalies are common. Inherited factors may play the predominant role in some patients.

The majority of patients cease to have convulsive equivalent attacks after puberty, but some may continue to have these attacks in adult life.

Autonomic and pain attacks of equivalent nature often respond quickly to Dilantin. Occasionally, it may be necessary to resort to other drugs, and of these Diamox and meprobamate have proved the most effective.

EXAMPLE: *Pain and Autonomic Equivalent*
            R. R., Clinic No. B-805

This boy, delivered by cesarean section because of placenta previa, was cyanotic at birth. A supernumerary thumb was present on the left hand and was later removed.

Clumsiness and smallness of the left side of his body were first noted when he was 6 months of age. Otherwise his development seemed normal.

At 6 months the child began to have episodes once or twice a week, in which he suddenly screamed as if in pain and held his head. About a minute after the onset he fell asleep and remained asleep and unresponsive for several hours. As he grew older the attack pattern changed. His mother noted that for an hour or so before an attack he was less active than usual. He then complained of epigastric pain and a bifrontal severe pounding headache. He sometimes vomited. If the attack was severe, the child might giggle without apparent provocation. After about a minute he lost consciousness, developed goose flesh and often fever up to 104° F. He slept, usually for two to three hours, and on awakening felt well except for occasional sensations of warmth or cold.

He had other attacks, occurring several times daily, in which he had epigastric pain for as long as 30 minutes. He often had headache at the same time.

When the child was examined at 7 years, his intelligence was estimated as superior. His left limbs were moderately small (hemiatrophy) and very slightly weak. His gait was abnormal because of shortness of his left lower limb.

An electroencephalogram at 7 years showed the pattern of 14 and 6 per second positive spikes in sleep (fig. 11). Dilantin and Mebaral were given and the patient was free of seizures for 12 months, the duration of his follow-up period.

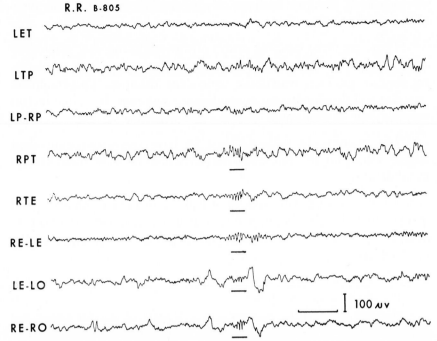

R.R. B-805

LET

LTP

LP-RP

RPT

RTE

RE-LE

LE-LO

100 ᴧᴠ

RE-RO

Figure 11. A 14 per second positive spike discharge is underlined in this figure. These positive spikes are usually of maximal amplitude in the posterior temporal region, but appear in the temporal and occipital leads.

Comment

With the exception of the loss of consciousness, all of the phenomena in these attacks—the vomiting, temperature alteration, pilo-erection, headache and epigastric pain—represent paroxysmal dysfunction in the autonomic centers. The 14 and 6 per second positive spike pattern is found in a high percentage of such cases, often in the absence of any other EEG abnormality. A good response to medication is usual.

REFERENCES

1. Klingman, W. O., Langford, W. S., Greeley, D. M. and Hoefer, P. F. A.: Paroxysmal attacks of abdominal pain, an epileptic equivalent in children. Tr. Am. Neurol. A., 67:228, 1941.

2. Hoefer, P. F. A., Cohen, S. M. and Greeley, D. M.: Paroxysmal abdominal pain, a form of epilepsy in children. J.A.M.A., 147:1, 1951.

3. Livingston, S.: Abdominal pain as a manifestation of epilepsy in children. J. Pediat., 38:687, 1951.

4. Gibbs, E. L. and Gibbs, F. A.: Electroencephalographic evidence of thalamic and hypothalamic epilepsy. Neurology, 1:136, 1951.

5. Mulder, D. W., Daly, D. and Bailey, A. A.: Visceral epilepsy. Arch. Int. Med., 93:481, 1954.

6. Heyck, H. and Hess, R.: Vasomotorische Kopfschmerzen als Symptom larvierter Epilepsien. Schweiz. med. Wchnschr., 85:573, 1955.

7. Kempton, J. J.: The periodic syndrome. Brit. M. J., 1:83, 1956.

8. O'Brien, J. L. and Goldensohn, E. S.: Paroxysmal abdominal pain as a manifestation of epilepsy. Neurology, 7:549, 1957.

9. Druckman, R.: Pain and autonomic disturbances in convulsive equivalent states. M. Clin. North America, 42:475, 1958.

10. Snyder, C. H.: Epileptic equivalents in children. Pediatrics, 21:308, 1958.

CHAPTER 9

Benign Febrile Convulsions
(B.F.C.)

IT HAS been estimated that about 5 per cent of unselected children in "well baby" clinics at one time or another have a convulsion. About 40 per cent of these, or about 2 to 3 per cent of all children, have seizures in association with fever. It is thus apparent that in children, and especially in young children, fever may precipitate a seizure. However, the important clinical fact here is that there is a group of young children who have particularly low thresholds to fever and who have seizures whenever their temperature goes beyond a certain point, this point being considerably below that at which the average child convulses. It is this group which constitutes the clinical entity of benign febrile convulsions, hereafter referred to as B.F.C. However, it should not be forgotten that fever is a non-specific precipitant of seizures and may activate seizures in children who have idiopathic or symptomatic epilepsy.

There is an important genetic factor in B.F.C. Statistical studies of patients with febrile convulsions have indicated a high familial incidence of seizures, varying in different reports from 20 to 50 per cent, figures which are greater than for any other type of seizure.

The great majority of children with B.F.C. do not develop chronic, recurrent, nonfebrile convulsions. The differentiation of B.F.C. from seizures likely to develop into chronic, recurrent epilepsy is an important feature of diagnosis in the child presenting with an initial febrile attack; a significant number of patients with chronic, nonfebrile, recurrent seizures, idiopathic or symptomatic, have their initial seizure triggered by fever. The possibility that the infection causing the fever involves the brain directly (meningoencephalitis) is a primary diagnostic consideration, particularly in infancy, and this possibility must be ruled out before a diagnosis of B.F.C. is made.

Several factors are helpful in differentiating B.F.C. from idiopathic or symptomatic epilepsy. These must be considered in their entirety in the evaluation of the patient:

(1) If the age of onset is between 6 months and 3 years, the seizures are more likely to be benign. An onset before 6 months of age suggests the probability of an underlying lesion of the brain as the likely cause of the seizure, with a consequently poorer outlook. After 3 years of age the seizures are likely to be idiopathic or symptomatic epilepsy, and are merely triggered by the fever.

(2) A slight elevation of temperature (less than 103° F.) occurring with seizures is more likely to be a sign that there is an underlying chronic convulsive disorder, rather than an indication of B.F.C.

(3) Well lateralized or focal seizures indicate the probability of a local cortical epileptogenic lesion (symptomatic epilepsy).

(4) The presence of abnormal neurological signs must be considered suggestive evidence of symptomatic epilepsy, rather than of B.F.C.

(5) A normal electroencephalogram favors a diagnosis of B.F.C., but this criterion is less reliable the younger the child. If abnormality is present in the EEG, the patient is then much more likely to develop chronic epilepsy. It is important, however, that the EEG be made after a sufficient time has elapsed following the seizure, so that any effects of the fever or of the seizure itself have subsided. A week is a safe interval.

(6) B.F.C. is more likely when there is a history that other members of the family were subject to the same type of attack.

Brain Damage As a Sequel of Febrile Convulsions

An important consideration in febrile convulsions is the possible development of brain damage as a result of the seizures themselves. This hazard becomes greater the more prolonged, severe or frequent are the attacks. Indications of brain injury may be transient or permanent. Findings such as transient hemiparesis following seizures (Todd's paralysis) indicate a reversible degree of cerebral injury. Permanent impairment of function may occur also, and the permanent injury may occur after there have been episodes of transient dysfunction. Even when the residual deficit is permanent, the immediately postictal impairment is usually much greater than the final functional loss.

The mechanism of the brain impairment following a seizure has not been established. Any prolonged seizure associated with cyanosis involves cerebral anoxia, which, combined with other unknown factors, may cause destruction or impairment of nerve cells. It has been proposed that a functional exhaustion can occur in the seizure, severe enough to lead to destruction of nerve cells, and that this loss of nerve cells may be either focal or diffuse. Another theory suggests that circulatory stasis in the convulsion predisposes to arterial thrombosis, with resulting cerebral damage; this is the cause of focal neurological deficits, such as hemiplegia. Perhaps one or another or several mechanisms may operate at different times. Also, there is a possibility that metabolic factors may have a role here. The raised metabolic rate associated with elevation of temperature increases the nutritional requirements of the nerve cells, and this increased demand makes the nerve cells more liable to injury by the excessive demand of the seizure discharge. Toxic substances secondary to the infectious process may also play a role in reducing the resistance of nerve cells to injury.

The most widely recognized sequel of febrile convulsions is a transient hemiparesis (Todd's paralysis). Permanent paralysis also can occur. It is probable, however, that more subtle changes in brain function are more common, such as behavorial disturbances, disorders of speech, mental retardation and chronic seizures. These latter developments, circumstantially at least, appear to be caused by the severe or prolonged febrile seizures. The electroencephalogram may provide confirmatory evidence of brain damage by the presence, for example, of a slow wave focus.

Treatment

If the patient is still convulsing when seen, it is obvious that anti-convulsant measures (as outlined in the treatment of status epilep-ticus, p. 125) should be instituted. Usually the patient has stopped convulsing when first seen; in this case the measures to be insti-tuted include cooling of the patient and the administration of salicyl-ates, if hyperpyrexia is present, and the use of antibiotics to eliminate any infection. Anticonvulsant medication should be given until the fever and infection clear. The drugs of choice are Dilantin or Mebaral (see the Drug Table, p. 138).

The course of further management depends on the diagnosis. Obviously, the treatment in any individual case will depend on the decision as to whether the problem is one of B.F.C. or one in which the fever was merely an activator of an underlying chronic convulsive disorder. For example, a child of 3 6/12 years with one convulsion brought on by low fever is more deserving of continuing treatment than is a patient of 18 months who has had two convulsions with high fever, because the probability of chronic recurrent epilepsy is greater in the former. If the circumstances and findings lead to a working diagnosis of B.F.C., the course of treatment is influenced by the number of seizures the patient has had. If the seizure is the first attack the child has experienced, no treatment is immediately instituted. However, instruction is given that the child be given antipyretics when fever threatens, and if fever continues to rise, cold sponging and ice packs should be used. The importance of seeking medical help earlier than is generally necessary when there is an onset of fever is stressed. If there is a history of more than one attack, anticonvulsant medication is begun, preferably with Dilantin, and continued for a period of not less than a year. Experience has shown that this procedure greatly reduces the risk of further seizures, and the protection thus gained against the possibility of brain im-pairment in seizures far outweighs any consideration against giving such medication.

The possible development of permanent brain damage in a very severe and prolonged febrile convulsion is the consideration that leads to the continuous use of anticonvulsant medication. Since infection may come on quickly in infants and not give any indica-tion of its presence until the seizure occurs, it is evident that sporadic administration of anticonvulsants at only those periods when the patient has an obvious infection or temperature elevation is not fully satisfactory. Thus, continuing treatment is likely to prove more effective than intermittent medication in preventing recurrences of seizures.

If a patient has had more than one febrile convulsion, he should have further studies, particularly electroencephalography. If a patient with febrile convulsions develops afebrile seizures, he should be managed along the lines laid down in the section on the general treatment of epilepsy.

EXAMPLE: *Benign Febrile Convulsions*
W.J.L., Clinic No. B-946

This girl was 1 9/12 years of age when she developed an upper respiratory and ear infection with fever. Two days after the onset of the infection she had a seizure which was generalized and lasted 10 minutes. Her temperature was reduced by cold sponges. That same night she had another similar seizure. About four weeks later she developed a sore throat, with an ear infection, fever and a convulsion. This time the convulsion started soon after the fever rose. This seizure was also generalized.

There was no family history of convulsive disorder.

When the patient was examined at 2 8/12 years of age, no abnormality was found. Laboratory investigation, including EEG, showed normal findings. The diagnosis was benign febrile convulsions; Dilantin, 25 mg. three times daily, was prescribed. The patient had no further seizures over the next two years. Repeat EEG showed no abnormality. The Dilantin was then reduced slowly to nil over three months, and the patient had no seizures for a further three months, the duration of the follow-up period.

REFERENCES

1. Lennox, W. G.: Significance of febrile convulsions. Pediatrics, 11:341, 1953.
2. Lennox, M. A.: Febrile convulsions in childhood. A. Research Nerv. and Ment. Dis., Proc., 26:342, 1947.
3. Schmidt, R. P. and Ward, A. A.: Febrile convulsions. Epilepsia, 4:41, 1955.
4. Prichard, J. S. and McGreal, D. A.: Febrile convulsions. M. Clin. North America, 42:379, 1958.

Breath-Holding Attacks

IT IS NOT uncommon for an infant to hold his breath in a bout of crying, but the majority of infants do this for only a brief period and that is all there is to the episode. However, a small number lose consciousness during these episodes, and it is with this group that the following discussion is concerned.

Breath-holding attacks as a clinical entity are those attacks which may be characterized as follows: In response to a painful experience the child begins to cry, suddenly holds his breath, becomes limp or stiff and loses consciousness. Some cyanosis of the lips and nails may be evident. Generally, the child remains either limp or rigid for a brief period and then quickly regains consciousness and appears normal. Occasionally, the rigid phase may be followed by a series of jerks or a typical tonic-clonic generalized seizure. Following any of these types of attacks the baby may fall asleep or be sleepy for a variable period. Breath-holding spells characteristically start between 6 and 12 months of age.

These attacks, by definition, occur only on provocation. The most frequent precipitant is an emotional upset, usually frustration. Sudden unexpected injury, no matter how slight, especially to the head, is a potent triggering agent. The actual holding of the breath

71

seldom lasts longer than 30 seconds and is usually much briefer, although parents often report its durations in terms of minutes. If a generalized seizure ensues, the attack may last for several minutes, but it is rarely as prolonged as this.

Breath holding is a disorder seen in otherwise normal children. The physical examination seldom reveals abnormality. The electro-encephalogram is normal between attacks but shows generalized slowing at the onset of unconsciousness. It is common to find a history of similar attacks in the patient's relatives.

The mechanism by which the loss of consciousness occurs in these breath-holding attacks has not been established. It seems unlikely that simple uncomplicated respiratory arrest with resulting anoxemia could bring about as rapid a loss of consciousness as occurs in these spells. As it is impossible to hold the breath to the point of unconsciousness voluntarily, it must be assumed that these patients have a defect or perhaps an exaggerated sensitivity of the mechanism which is involved in the transient reflex apnea (gasp) induced by a sudden fright. Some believe that altered intrathoracic pressures sharply reduce the cardiac output with resultant cerebral ischemia and loss of consciousness in these attacks. There is also a psychogenic factor involved, in that the attacks are more common in spoiled children who have overprotective, oversolicitous parents.

There is another type of attack which appears to be closely related to breath-holding spells, in that it occurs in response to a sudden "noxious" stimulus. In these attacks, the breath-holding component is not present and the effective stimulus, usually a blow to the head, will produce immediate unconsciousness. The pain of injury does not need to be severe, and a comparatively mild blow may produce the effect as easily as a sharp one.

The criteria for differentiating breath-holding spells from epilepsy are: (1) The necessary presence of a provoking stimulus, and (2) an onset with a sudden holding of the breath.

Breath-holding attacks are a benign syndrome, and the attacks usually cease spontaneously by 2 to 3 years of age. Generally, there are no residual effects but rarely, if the attacks are numerous and prolonged, brain damage from anoxia may result. There is no convincing evidence that breath-holding spells predispose to the later development of epilepsy; the number of children with this type of spell who develop chronic epilepsy is not significantly greater than the incidence of epilepsy in the general population.

Treatment of children with breath-holding spells requires that the parents be informed of the benign nature of the attacks. They should be instructed not to appear too concerned over these spells, since it is clear that these attacks, once started, may become an attention-getting or manipulative mechanism. Our experience indicates that medication is useful in these patients. Dilantin has proved the most effective of the drugs tested, but Mebaral and chlorpromazine are also sometimes helpful. Drug treatment is given for the following reasons: (1) Reduction in the frequency of attacks may be achieved, (2) reduction in the likelihood that the attacks will be complicated by convulsive movements, and (3) more important, the reduction of the possibility of brain damage from anoxia. Drug treatment is continued for about a year.

EXAMPLE: *Breath-Holding Attacks*
          C.F., Clinic No. B-736

At 1 year of age this girl began to cry after fright or injury, hold her breath, become blue about the face and lips and then fall unconscious. Her eyes became glassy and her body rigid for a few seconds and she then became limp. These spells usually occurred about every two months, but often recurred every week. The usual precipitants were sudden frights or mild injuries, but occasionally the spells were brought on by temper tantrums; the most effective precipitant was unexpected bodily injury. There were frequent spells of breath holding without loss of consciousness.

The patient's birth history and developmental milestones were normal. A paternal grandfather was epileptic.

Examination at 2 6/12 years revealed no abnormality. Skull roentgenograms and the EEG showed nothing abnormal. Mebaral, 16 mg. three times daily, was prescribed. The breath-holding spells gradually became less frequent.

At 2 11/12 years of age, the child fell off a tricycle, made a sighing noise and was found unconscious by her mother. She still occasionally held her breath after crying hard but did not lose consciousness. At 3 6/12 years the medication was stopped. At 5 years of age the patient was doing well, without loss of consciousness and without breath holding for the last two years.

REFERENCES

1. Bridge, E. M., Livingston, S. and Tietze, C.: Breath-holding spells. J. Pediat., 23:539, 1943.
2. Low, N. L., Gibbs, E. L. and Gibbs, F. A.: Electroencephalographic findings in breath-holding spells. Pediatrics, 15:595, 1955.
3. (Lead article) Breath-holding attacks. Brit. M. J., 2:422, 1955.

CHAPTER II

Epilepsy of Adult Life

JUST AS the incidence of the various causes of seizures varies between the first few months of life and later childhood, so do the causes of seizures vary in different phases of adult life. There is practically no idiopathic epilepsy (as previously defined) with an onset after the age of 20 years. Indeed, the age of onset of seizures is a factor of prime consideration in determining the probable cause of the attacks. Between 20 and 40 years of age trauma is the major cause of seizures, with cerebral tumors following in second place. Between 40 and 60 years the most common cause of seizures is tumor, with trauma, vascular disease and neurosyphilis the next most common causes, in that order. From 60 years of age and above vascular cerebral disease is the leading cause of seizures, with cerebral tumors and degenerative diseases being less common.

Cerebrovascular Disease

Vascular disorder is the commonest cause of epilepsy of onset after 60 years. Atherosclerosis is the major condition and is often, though not necessarily, associated with hypertension. Only a minority of patients with cerebral arteriosclerosis show hardening of the peripheral vessels, but thickening of the retinal arterioles provides a better indication of the state of the cerebral arteries.

75

With arteriolosclerosis there are diffuse atrophic changes in the brain, while with hardening and thrombosis of larger arteries the brain lesions tend to be more focal. Seizures occur in about 20 per cent of those with autopsy findings of cerebrovascular disease. Generalized vascular disease of the brain is about three times commoner than is purely focal infarction. Seizures accompany or follow cerebral infarction or cerebral hemorrhage in about 12 per cent of cases. Only half of this group have recurrent seizures, and these seizures tend to have focal characteristics. Chronic epilepsy may be the only residual clinical manifestation of a stroke.

Hypertensive encephalopathy is an occasional cause of seizures. The diagnosis is based upon the severe hypertension with its associated retinal changes and on the common occurrence of repeated transient neurological deficits.

Embolism, secondary to endocarditis or auricular fibrillation, is another cause of cerebral infarction and seizures. Polyarteritis nodosa and cerebral thromboangiitis obliterans are rare vascular disorders which, when they involve the brain, can produce seizures.

Trauma

Traumatic brain damage may occur as a result of penetrating wounds or of head injury without penetration of the dura. Most studies of this problem are based on the incidence of epilepsy following war injuries. The longer the follow-up period, the higher is the incidence of seizures. About 45 per cent of gunshot wounds with penetration of the dura are followed by epilepsy, while the incidence of seizures is half this when there is no penetration of the dura. Sepsis increases the likelihood of later epilepsy. Epileptogenic scars may be cerebrodural or involve only cortical tissue without meningeal participation in the scar.

Seizures may appear within a few days of injury and then cease permanently, or the onset of post-traumatic attacks might be months to years following the initial injury and be chronically recurrent.

Tumors

Epilepsy occurs in about 30 per cent of cerebral neoplasms, and it may provide the initial symptom of the tumor. There is a higher incidence of seizures in tumors located in the temporal, frontal and parietal regions than in occipital mass lesions. Seizures are slightly more frequent in gliomas than in meningomas.

Suspicion of cerebral neoplasm as the likely cause of seizures is high when the onset of seizures is between 35 and 50 years of age. However, such tumors are not likely to be present if the history or examination shows no evidence of progressive dysfunction or increased intracranial pressure. If, when the patient is first seen, the history of seizures dates back five or more years, then the likelihood of cerebral tumor as the cause of the convulsive disorder is small. If progressive deficit of function, abnormal neurological findings, evidence of focal electroencephalographic disturbance or abnormality on skull roentgenograms are present, the suspicion of cerebral neoplasm is increased and further investigation (by air study, angiograms or biopsy) is indicated.

Cerebral Infections

Syphilis of the brain, considerably less common now than previously, can be a cause of seizures; this possibility should not be forgotten, because of the importance of early institution of specific treatment. The seizures in general paresis are associated with other evidences of disturbed cerebral function, such as mental changes, slurred speech and tremor, and it is the prevention of irreversible cerebral deterioration which makes early recognition and treatment of this infection so important.

About 50 per cent of the patients with cerebral abscess have seizures. Seizures are most common with frontal abscesses, and the incidence of such attacks decreases with location in the parietal, temporal and occipital regions, in that order. The type of infecting organism does not influence the incidence of seizures. Attacks may occur both in the acute phase and following excision of the lesion.

If the diagnosis of cerebral abscess is made early, antibiotic therapy should be given to encourage encapsulation, for surgical excision before encapsulation increases the likelihood of seizures. About 75 per cent of patients with cerebral abscesses have had seizures within a year following the surgical excision of the abscess.

Pyogenic meningoencephalitis and viral encephalitis, though

less common in adults than in children, can also cause convulsions in the older age group. Parasitic brain infection (cysticercosis, hydatid cysts, malaria or schistosomiasis) are other rare causes of seizures.

Toxic Causes

Alcoholism is an important cause of cerebral deterioration and seizures in the adult. The brain damage may be caused by a toxic effect of alcohol or by associated nutritional deficiency, or by both. Frequently, head injuries incurred during intoxication are a factor in the development of a seizure state.

Upon sudden withdrawal from their source of drug, barbiturate addicts may develop severe convulsions.

Miscellaneous

DEGENERATIVE CEREBRAL DISORDERS

Seizures may occur in association with mental deterioration in Alzheimer's and Pick's diseases. These disorders are rare and seizures are incidental, the dementia being the predominant feature of these conditions.

MALFORMATIONS

Seizures may appear in adult life and yet be secondary to congenital cerebral defects (for example, angiomatous malformations), but the usual onset of seizures of this causation is in childhood.

DEMYELINATING DISEASE

It has been estimated that about 3 per cent of patients with multiple sclerosis develop seizures. In these instances seizures are usually much less troublesome than the other neurological deficits and usually occur in the later stages of the illness or with sudden exacerbations of the disease.

REFERENCES

1. Walker, A. E.: Convulsive seizures in adult life. Arch. Int. Med., 58:250, 1936.
2. White, P. T., Bailey, A. A. and Bickford, R. G.: Epileptic disorders in the aged. Neurology, 3:674, 1953.

3. Dodge, P. R., Richardson, E. P. and Victor, M.: Recurrent convulsive seizures as a sequel to cerebral infarction: a clinical and pathological study.
   Brain, 77:610, 1954.

4. Northcroft, G. B. and Wyke, B. D.: Seizures following surgical treatment of
   intracranial abscesses (a clinical and electroencephalographic study).
   J. Neurosurg., 14:249, 1957.

5. Denny-Brown, D.: The clinical aspects of traumatic epilepsy. Am. J. Psychiat., 100:585, 1944.

6. Watson, C. W.: Incidence of epilepsy following craniocerebral injury; three
   year follow-up study. Arch. Neurol. and Psychiat., 68:831, 1952.

7. Dimsdale, H.: Epilepsy of late onset in the light of modern diagnostic procedures. Brit. M. J., 1:1214, 1956.

CHAPTER 12

Extracerebral Factors in Convulsions

LOSS OF consciousness and convulsions sometimes occur as a result of factors which are essentially extracerebral. In such, the seizures are produced by a transient effect upon the brain by primary metabolic or circulatory systemic disturbances. The extracerebral disorders which most commonly cause seizures are hypoglycemia, syncope, the Stokes-Adams syndrome, congenital cyanotic heart disease, uremia and hypocalcemia.

Hypoglycemia

Hypoglycemia may cause attacks of unconsciousness and convulsions. Such attacks usually come on several hours after the ingestion of food. Premonitory symptoms of hunger, faintness, weakness, perspiration and nausea are the rule. The patient may then become confused and lapse into unconsciousness. Convulsions may supervene. The blood sugar level at which symptoms occur is usually between 20 to 40 mg. per cent, although diabetic patients may show symptoms and signs at higher blood sugar levels. Administration of food is generally sufficient to abort an attack. Once stupor has supervened it may be necessary to give intravenous glucose.

Hypoglycemic episodes of this severity are most frequently seen following an overdosage of insulin in diabetic patients. When such attacks occur spontaneously in patients who are not diabetic, tumors or hyperplasia of the islet cells of the pancreas or severe liver damage (e.g., glycogen storage disease) may be possible causes. Fasting blood sugar, glucose tolerance, insulin sensitivity and liver function tests should be carried out to determine the basic cause.

If prolonged coma occurs in the hypoglycemic episodes, permanent damage to the brain may result.

In the diagnosis of hyperinsulinism, a flat glucose tolerance curve with low values at two and one-half hours and beyond is helpful. An insulin sensitivity test, in which insulin is administered in a given amount and the response of the blood sugar curve measured, is the most useful laboratory procedure in the diagnosis of islet cell hyperfunction. A low blood sugar during or immediately following a seizure or an attack of unconsciousness, and a dramatic response to the administration of glucose are practically diagnostic of hypoglycemia. The electroencephalogram in normoglycemic periods is normal, but shows during the premonitory phase and during the attack itself progressive slowing and the development of paroxysmal slow activity. The presence of other types of abnormality, such as generalized spike and wave bursts or focal abnormality, throws doubt on a diagnosis of hypoglycemia. However, the electrical activity accompanying the convulsive seizure is indistinguishable from that seen in other generalized true tonic-clonic seizures of any cause.

Treatment involves providing orange juice or candy for the immediate attack, and reducing the insulin dosage when hypoglycemia is due to overdosage of insulin. Recently, cortisone has been successfully used in the treatment of idiopathic hypoglycemia, but extirpation is indicated for islet cell adenoma.

The particular premonitory symptoms described above and their disappearance with ingestion of sugar helps to differentiate these attacks from epilepsy. The term "epilepsy" should not be applied to hypoglycemic episodes, since it, by definition, refers to seizures of primarily intracerebral origin. It should be noted that convulsive attacks due entirely to hypoglycemia are comparatively rare, but even relatively mild hypoglycemia may precipitate seizures in patients with epilepsy.

Hypocalcemia

Rarely, patients with hypocalcemia have convulsions as a direct effect of this disturbance of ionic equilibrium. However, scattered muscle twitchings occurring in hypocalcemia should be differentiated from true convulsions, since the former are of peripheral rather than cerebral origin. These twitchings are generally random and scattered and may be precipitated by various stimuli, such as loud sounds and movement.

The blood calcium level must fall below about 7 mg. per cent and the product of the concentrations of calcium and of phosphorous must fall below 40 before such symptoms supervene. Rickets, celiac disease, hypoparathyroidism, pseudohypoparathyroidism and severe vomiting may produce hypocalcemia and symptoms which may be confused with epilepsy.

Intravenous calcium gluconate should be given at once and maintenance therapy with calcium chloride continued for some time in hypocalcemia. Sedation is also helpful. The cause of the basic metabolic defect should be discovered and corrected.

Uremia

Convulsions may occur in uremia. Some chemical changes are present, including the retention of phosphates, nitrogenous wastes, sodium, potassium and water, but it is uncertain which of these factors or combinations of factors serve to produce the seizures. Scattered twitchings without loss of consciousness also occur, but these are quite easily distinguished from convulsions.

Toxic Causes

In acute seizures of the generalized tonic-clonic type, the possibility of intoxication should be considered. Children commonly ingest insecticides (alkyl phosphate sprays), hydrocarbon solvents, lead, thallium and salicylates in sufficient quantities to produce an acute convulsive state.

The character of the associated symptoms varies with the poison to which the patient has been exposed, but the following factors may be helpful in suggesting the diagnosis of intoxication: a sudden onset of vomiting or drowsiness, any unusual odor or the possession of a bottle or other container in which poisons or drugs had been kept.

Toxic states are often completely reversible, and immediate and proper treatment may control seizures and prevent the development of a persistent encephalopathy. Once the diagnosis is established, treatment should be directed first to the removal of the poison by stomach lavage, if ingestion has been by mouth, or by other methods appropriate to the type of poison and its route of absorption. Anticonvulsant drugs should be given as soon as possible for the control of seizures. If respiration is depressed, the barbiturates should be avoided and paraldehyde or hydantoinates used.

Cardiovascular Causes

Disturbed function of the brain, manifest in loss of consciousness or in convulsions, may be secondary to a transient inadequacy of the blood supply to the brain. This occurs when the cardiac output is diminished, whether because of decreased venous return to the heart as in syncope, or as a result of cardiac dysrhythmia as in the Stokes-Adams syndrome, tachycardias and carotid sinus hypersensitivity.

Syncope (Fainting)

In true syncope the patient becomes dizzy, weak and pale and has a feeling of faintness. He then falls unconscious and remains so for a relatively brief period. This is a vasomotor phenomenon which may result from emotional shock, from orthostatic hypotension or from carotid sinus activation. By definition, syncope is not associated with convulsive movements. The recumbent position is sufficient to restore the blood supply to the brain so that consciousness returns before the ischemia is sufficient to produce a convulsion.

Stokes-Adams Syndrome

The cerebral ischemia which occurs in heart block as a result of ventricular arrest may lead to loss of consciousness, transient tonic extension of the trunk and limbs or generalized convulsions, or combinations of any of these. Such attacks may be quite frequent, depending upon the incidence of the change from partial to complete heart block.

This disorder occurs mainly in older people and is most often due to arteriosclerotic heart disease. It can occur in young adults and children where myocarditis or congenital abnormalities of the conducting system are present. Rarely, paroxysmal ventricular tachycardia, of a degree sufficient to limit the cardiac output, may produce similar attacks.

CHAPTER 13

The Investigation of

Seizure Patients

A PREREQUISITE of proper treatment and prognostic evaluation of the seizure patient is the establishment of an accurate and
complete diagnosis. This requires first a thorough understanding of
the nature of the various convulsive states. A detailed history must
be obtained and a careful physical examination made. This might
appear obvious, but too often these aspects of investigation are
neglected and too much reliance is placed on laboratory studies.
The clinical information is always the most important factor in
evaluating the seizure patient, and usually in itself provides the essential evidence for diagnosis. Various laboratory tests, such as EEG,
skull roentgenograms, lumbar puncture, air encephalography and
angiography, may be employed where variously indicated to provide
adjunctive diagnostic information, such as the localization and the
nature of an underlying cerebral lesion.

The usefulness of the history depends upon the examiner's
ability to obtain from the patient information which will point to
the nature of his disorder. This ability, in turn, requires that the
physician have sufficient knowledge of the convulsive states so that

87

he is able to recognize the clues provided by the patient's story and to develop this information by asking pertinent questions, especially with regard to the features of the patient's attacks. The most subtle and often apparently improbable features of the patient's story may be important clues to the diagnosis. The questioning of the patient should be determined by the character and circumstances of the patient's complaints.

The first step in diagnosis is the determination of whether the patient's attacks are truly epileptic or due to extracerebral causes such as hypoglycemia. If it is decided that the patient is suffering from an epileptic disorder, the next diagnostic step is to establish whether the attacks are due to idiopathic or symptomatic epilepsy, and if symptomatic to determine the cause of the underlying cerebral lesion. If it is decided that the epilepsy is symptomatic in origin, the next, logical step is to determine whether the lesion is stationary (as in a cerebral scar) or progressive (as in a tumor). The questioning is then directed, if the lesion is static, toward determining the remote cause of the cerebral lesion. The common causes of symptomatic epilepsy are reviewed in chapter 5.

Abnormalities found on neurological examination, if referable to the brain, favor a symptomatic rather than an idiopathic epilepsy. The presumption is that the lesion responsible for the abnormal neurological findings is the cause of the cerebral seizures. The neurological abnormality may also provide clues to the localization of the lesion. For example, a spastic hemiparesis is indicative of a contralateral frontal lesion. A hemianopic field defect is usually indicative of a temporal or occipital lesion on the opposite side. Aphasia is an indication of a lesion of the dominant cerebral hemisphere, particularly of lesions involving the superior temporal and inferior frontal regions. A combination of right hemiparesis, homonymous hemianopia and aphasia would be indicative of a left deep frontotemporal lesion. Sensory defects, such as astereognosis, defective two-point discrimination and impaired position sense, are often traced to parietal lobe lesions. If the neurological localization corresponds with the localizing features of the aura, then there is good evidence that a single lesion is causing both the neurological abnormality and the epilepsy. Absence of neurological abnormality, however, does not rule out an underlying lesion. The presence of such may be established by laboratory findings or by the character of the seizures.

The findings of the general physical examination are often most helpful. For example, a vascular nevus of the face in a seizure patient suggests the possibility of a similar anomaly of the brain. Adenoma sebaceum makes the diagnosis of tuberous sclerosis likely. The association of a stiff neck and fever with convulsions indicates the possibility of meningoencephalitis. The general physical examination also may provide evidence which establishes that the seizures are due to a primarily systemic condition as, for example, collagen disease or hypertension.

The diagnostic impression derived from the history and physical examination should determine if there is any indication for laboratory studies and, if so, what these studies should be. The local availability and quality of such studies may be a further factor in such a decision. For example, an initial febrile seizure in a child may not require any laboratory studies if the presumptive diagnosis based on the history and physical examination is benign febrile convulsions. Conversely, laboratory studies are essential in a young adult with a first seizure and a history of progressive local weakness, in order to establish the character and localization of the causative lesion.

Of the various laboratory procedures used in the study of the epileptic patient, electroencephalography can be the most productive. Unfortunately, however, there is more variation from place to place in the reliability of this study than for other laboratory tests. EEG frequently provides the only objective evidence of cerebral disorder in seizure patients. It is also of great help in differentiating between diffuse cerebral dysfunction, such as occurs in encephalitis, from more localized disorders. It may help in localization and may provide evidence as to whether the lesion is static or progressive.

Roentgenographic examination of the skull occasionally provides unique information concerning seizure patients, but this test is revealing in a far smaller proportion of patients than is electroencephalography. Abnormal calcification may help localize a cerebral lesion, and the type of calcification may provide a clue to the nature of the underlying lesion. For example, characteristic patterns of calcification present in the Sturge-Weber syndrome permit an etiological diagnosis. The roentgenographic examination of the skull may also reveal indications of increased intracranial pressure, such as erosion of the dorsum sellae, and may thus direct the nature of further investigation.

EEG and skull films are generally required in patients with convulsive disorder. Each is a harmless and painless procedure, capable of providing information unobtainable by other means.

Lumbar puncture and examination of the cerebrospinal fluid is not mandatory in all seizure patients. It is of particular value when brain tumor or inflammatory disease is suspected and should be done in all cases of suspected progressive degenerative disease. There are, however, cases in which CSF studies are mandatory. It is essential, for instance, to do such studies in all cases in which meningitis is suspected. The results of the CSF examination may establish the nature of the disease and thus determine therapy. Because other evidence of inflammatory cerebral disease, such as stiffness of the neck or even fever, may be absent in the young infant, CSF studies should always be made in young infants who have an initial convulsion.

Pneumoencephalography is indicated where there is a possibility of cerebral tumor, but the decision to do this procedure should be tempered by the presence of increased intracranial pressure as indicated by papilledema, bulging fontanel, suture separation, erosion of the dorsum sellae and other conditions. Ventriculography may be the procedure of choice where there is evidence of increased intracranial pressure. Pneumoencephalography should be performed prior to surgical excision of epileptogenic lesions, for it may reveal evidence of further localizing value.

Angiograms may be of value where the history or physical examination suggests the possibility of an angiomatous malformation as, for example, in a case in which there have been recurrent unilateral headaches and subarachnoid hemorrhages. Angiography may reveal information of great value in cerebral tumors, for it may not only provide evidence relating to the localization of the expanding lesion, but the vascular pattern in the region of the lesion may suggest the nature of the tumor present.

Electrocorticography and depth recording are highly specialized procedures which are only employed where precise localization of an epileptogenic lesion is required prior to surgical extirpation. Electrocorticography is the technique of directly recording the electrical activity of the cerebral cortex by means of electrodes placed on the brain exposed at craniotomy. This is used to delimit discharging lesions of the convexity of the hemispheres and to ensure that all epileptogenic tissue has been removed. The reason that electrocorticography is necessary is that the abnormally discharging tissue may appear grossly normal, while the obvious lesion may not itself be the source of any abnormal activity (see the histopathology of brain scars, p. 11).

Depth recording is only necessary in cases in which the epileptogenic lesion is believed to lie in parts of the cerebral cortex or in other structures which are inaccessible to electrocorticography, such as the hippocampus. The electrodes are placed in the brain through small burr holes, and the technique has the advantage that the electrodes may be left in place for relatively long periods and recordings can be made over a period of days and even weeks. The procedure can be done without significant injury to the brain, and thus permits preoperative exploration in cases in which the exact localization of the lesion is problematic.

Blood chemistries need not be routinely required but should be carried out when the history suggests the possibility of metabolic disorder. For example, glucose tolerance tests are indicated where the history and seizure pattern are suggestive of hypoglycemic episodes. Serum calcium determinations are done much more often in practice than is really indicated, but they can provide useful information when hypocalcemia is a possibility. It is important to realize that the significant factor is the ionizable calcium rather than the total calcium content. Serum nonprotein nitrogen determination or blood urea nitrogen is necessary where there is a history of kidney disorder, because of the possibility that the seizures were precipitated by uremia. In rare cases of seizures associated with primary mental retardation, blood or urine testing may reveal an inborn metabolic defect, such as phenylketonuria.

The results of the history, physical examination and laboratory tests must be integrated into a meaningful whole in deciding the cause of the convulsive disorder. Accurate diagnosis, based on such a synthesis, determines appropriate therapy.

CHAPTER 14

Electroencephalography in the Diagnosis and Management of the Epilepsies

T HE ELECTROENCEPHALOGRAPH (fig. 12) is essentially an instrument designed to amplify the electrical activity of the brain to a point at which it can be recorded by a suitable ink-writing or similar device upon a moving chart. In order to make it possible to record from several parts of the head at one time and so that the activity from each side of the brain can be simultaneously compared, several amplifiers are used. The number of individual amplifiers, or "channels," in a given piece of apparatus varies, but modern usage usually requires from six to eight channels. Each amplifier is connected to the head by means of a pair of electrodes, consisting of a small metal cup made of silver, lead or similar metal, and attached to a short length of wire. These are attached to the head with a special paste which is highly conductive, and are held in place by tape, paraffin, collodion or some other adhesive material (fig. 13, A). The number of electrodes applied to the skull varies in different

93

laboratories, but minimum coverage requires that a placement be made on each side over the frontal, parietal, occipital and temporal lobes and that a common reference electrode be employed on each of the ears or elsewhere at a distance from the brain (fig. 13, B and C). When the brain abnormality is of a focal character, extra electrodes may be employed in order to define more closely the locus of the lesion.

The method most commonly used in this country is based on the idea that the best way to record is to have one electrode (of each channel) at a point distant from the brain,* and thus electrically silent. The activity then picked up, theoretically, would be simply that arising directly under the other electrode located on the scalp. The ear lobes are commonly used as the indifferent point for the reference electrode in this so-called "monopolar" technique. However, because of the proximity of the ears to the temporal lobes, such electrodes may pick up activity of brain origin, especially if there is abnormality in this region; therefore, these are not always truly "indifferent."

The other method is the simple one of recording between any two electrodes on the scalp itself. This is the so-called "scalp to scalp" or "bipolar" technique and it essentially records the sum of the electrical activity occurring simultaneously under each of the two electrodes selected.

Ideally, the patient should be placed in a quiet room on a bed remote from the electroencephalographic machine and the recording activities. This is necessary both for the relaxation and comfort of the patient during the long recording period often required, and also for the purpose of encouraging sleep, which is often an effective activator of epileptic abnormality.

The fact that abnormality may appear in the electroencephalograms of epileptic patients in the interseizure period is the very basis of clinical electroencephalographic studies; but, because epileptic abnormalities are, by their very character, sporadic or paroxysmal, relatively long periods of recording are generally required for the adequate study of patients suspected of having epilepsy. However, the tendency for such abnormality to appear spontaneously is subject

* Unfortunately, it is not practical to place an "indifferent" electrode very far away because of pick-up of the electrical activity of the heart, a much higher voltage electrical signal.

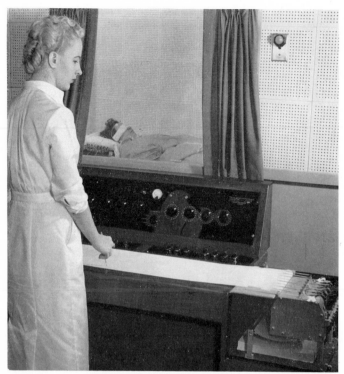

Figure 12. A recording unit of the EEG Department, Methodist Hospital, Houston, Texas. Note that the patient is in a room separate from the recording activities and is reclining on a bed. The electroencephalograph shown is an eight channel Offner, Type D.

to considerable variation from patient to patient and, in some instances, abnormality may not appear at all unless evoked by some special procedure. The simplest of these is the use of sleep, which has been demonstrated to be a potent activator of latent abnormalities in patients with convulsive disorders. In order to obtain sleep, it is often necessary to use mild sedation, and this has become routine in many laboratories. Occasionally, intravenous hypnotic or anesthetic doses of barbiturates or similar drugs are employed, but this is generally not as productive. Oral administration of a sedative dose of a fast-acting barbiturate or, in the case of infants, the use of a barbiturate suppository generally suffices to produce sleep if the conditions are otherwise conducive.

Hyperventilation, or overbreathing, for periods of about three minutes, is employed routinely by most laboratories to bring out

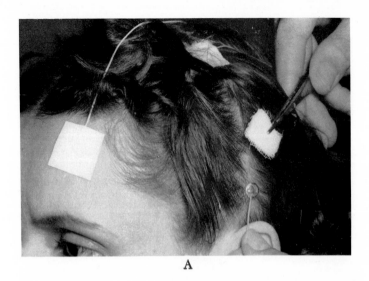

A

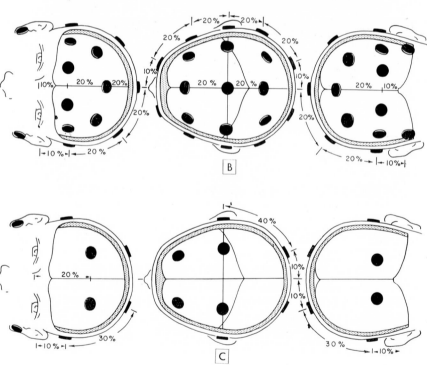

Figure 13. (A) Attachment of the electrode. The silver disk electrode with its connecting wire is in place in the temporal area and is sticking to the skin by the bentonite paste beneath it. The square of gauze, which has been dipped in paraffin wax of low melting temperature, is about to be placed over

latent convulsive activity and to test the general reactivity of the brain to low carbon dioxide levels. The paroxysmal generalized spike and wave discharge of idiopathic epilepsy is, for example, particularly liable to activation by this procedure. Epileptics in general have been demonstrated to show a more marked and persistent lability to low carbon dioxide levels in the blood than do normal controls.*

In problem cases in which these "physiologic" methods of activation fail to reveal evidence of abnormality, resort may be made to chemical activation. Metrazol has been the most commonly used agent for this purpose. This drug, when administered intravenously, will often activate focal epileptogenic lesions of the brain and produce electroencephalographic abnormality in the region of the lesion. Careful control of the rate of administration in relationship to the changes that are taking place in the electroencephalogram usually is sufficient to prevent the onset of a clinical seizure. Paroxysmal generalized 3 per second waves or abortive spike and wave responses to Metrazol are probably nonspecific, as they may be elicited at low dosages in normal individuals, and only focal responses can be considered diagnostically reliable findings.

What Does the Electroencephalograph Record?

Simply stated, the electroencephalogram performs the same duty as an electrocardiogram, in that it records electrical activity from the organ which is being studied. In the case of the heart, this electrical activity is coming from a more or less homogeneous structure.

* This is the electroencephalographic factor most commonly misinterpreted. Big build-ups of slow activity are commonly seen in normal children, and conservative evaluation of overbreathing responses should always be made, especially in the young child.

---

the electrode to hold it firmly to the skin and hair. The hair does not have to be cut with this method; it is necessary only to clean the skin first by rubbing with ether-acetone mixture. An electrode is shown attached to the parietal area by this method. The electrode in the frontal area is held in place by a square of orthopedic tape, since this is a better method for hair-free areas. (B) The position of the recording electrodes as standardized by the International Electroencephalographic Society. The position of each placement is determined by the percentage of distance between nasion and inion in the longitudinal plane (10–20 system), and between the external auditory meati in the transverse or coronal plane. (C) The minimal number of electrode placements for routine electrographic studies.

In the case of the brain, it is arising from millions of individual neurons which do not behave as a homogeneous whole, but which are capable, to some extent, of independent activity. It is important to realize that this electrical activity is generated by each individual cell of the brain and that it represents an essential element of the life process or metabolism of these cells. When the function of the neurons is impaired, so, too, is the electrical activity impaired or distorted.

Because the electrodes are placed on the surface of the skull, the activity which is recorded in routine electroencephalography is essentially that of the cerebral cortex. However, because the cortex is itself under the influence of subcortical structures, lesions which impair or alter the activity of subcortical structures may, nevertheless, be reflected in the electrical activity of the cortex and thus in the simple electroencephalogram as recorded from the scalp; this makes possible diagnosis and evaluation of epilepsies which have their origin in the deep central structures of the brain, particularly the thalamus.

Application of Electroencephalography

Electroencephalography provides a harmless and painless method of evaluating patients with known or suspected cerebral abnormalities. There are no contraindications to its use, except where extensive wounds of the scalp may make it impractical because of possible infection. The technique does not require extensive or particular preparation of the patient. Generally, all that is required is that the patient's scalp be clean and free of oil and, for this reason, instruction is often given for the hair to be washed prior to recording. No dietary requirements are usually necessary and, in fact, adequate meals should be taken prior to the test, since normal blood sugar levels are desirable. Stimulating beverages, such as coffee and tea, should, of course, be avoided if a sleep study is to be made.

The question often asked by practitioners is, "When should an electroencephalogram be obtained?" The answer to this question is, of course, complicated by the limited availability of facilities for recording electroencephalograms and the scarcity of trained electroencephalographers to interpret them. Ideally, however, electroencephalographic studies should be made in all patients in whom convulsive disorder is known to exist or is suspected on clinical grounds. In the first instance, clinical diagnosis is always limited in its certainty by the fact that the physician rarely witnesses the attacks and is dependent so often upon the reporting of witnesses, who, because of the dramatic course of events, may not be able to give a coherent or complete description. Furthermore, the differential diagnosis of certain of the focal epilepsies from seizures which are of idiopathic origin often is not possible without the aid of an electroencephalogram. Since generalized seizures may arise both in symptomatic and idiopathic epilepsy, and may even occur in patients with focal lesions of the brain, the electroencephalogram is often essential in making a differential diagnostic evaluation of the patient with a generalized seizure as the sole presenting symptom.

The factor of age is, to some extent, a consideration in this problem. An initial febrile convulsion in an infant might not be considered cause to send a patient to a distant center for electroencephalographic study, while an initial convulsion in a 40 year old man, even in the absence of other abnormality, might certainly be a strong indication that such a step was necessary.

The Proper Role of Electroencephalography in the Total Evaluation of the Patient

The electroencephalogram should not be considered a means of obtaining a "penny in the slot" diagnosis. Electroencephalography does, however, provide an insight into the patient which is not otherwise obtainable; namely, a picture of the functioning of the brain as it is reflected at the cortex in electrical terms. This activity is rarely diagnostic in itself, but when evaluated in relation to the clinical history and findings, it may facilitate the development of a total factual pattern which makes diagnosis possible. A simple example of the necessity for understanding the importance of correlating clinical and electroencephalographic findings in order to obtain diagnosis is illustrated by the relatively common (approximately 12 per cent) finding of a normal electroencephalogram in patients known to have seizures. Obviously, it would be ridiculous in the face of recurrent generalized tonic-clonic seizures to claim that this patient was normal because he had a normal electroencephalogram. Similarly, it would be equally ridiculous to claim that a patient known to have a single seizure and referred for diagnostic study was not epileptic because his electroencephalogram was normal. Because epilepsy is, by nature, a paroxysmal disturbance of brain function, it is possible for the electroencephalograph of some patients to be normal in interseizure periods. Fortunately, when all simple activation techniques are employed, such as overventilation and sleep, the number of such patients is reduced to a maximum of about 8 per cent. Conversely, the existence of definite epileptiform patterns as, for example, paroxysmal 3 per second spike and wave discharge, in a patient should not be considered evidence per se that this patient has clinical epilepsy. The electrical pattern merely indicates that the neuronal storms which are the basis of epilepsy are present in the brain. The outward or overt manifestations may not necessarily have occurred.

Thus, the correct or rational use of electroencephalography is as an adjunct to clinical evaluation, providing a means of insight into the patient which is not otherwise obtainable, but by no means providing a magic key to total diagnosis. This consideration brings out another factor which is important in the effective clinical use of electroencephalography. A single study, no matter how complete, is often insufficient in certain problem patients. Thus, two or more studies at different times may be required to demonstrate the presence of abnormality. A good example of this is in cases of "abdominal" epilepsy, in which it is sometimes necessary to resort to recording at the time of an attack in order to demonstrate the change in the patient's brain waves. But here, certainly, the extra trouble of obtaining records under these circumstances is worth the diagnosis that might not otherwise be made.

Electroencephalographic Abnormalities and Their Clinical Correlates

As mentioned before, the electrencephalogram should be used to provide adjunctive information in order to arrive at a final diagnosis. The electroencephalogram rarely provides specific diagnostic patterns which, in themselves, tell the whole or even a large part of the story. Electroencephalographic findings are, in this way, comparable to the findings of electrocardiography. The electroencephalogram never provides *all* the information necessary for diagnosis. However, there are certain specific electrographic patterns, the significance of which has been clearly established, which provide definite clues to the differential evaluation of the patient's disorder.

3 PER SECOND SPIKE AND WAVE PATTERNS

Perhaps the most reliably specific electroencephalographic abnormality is that known as the 3 per second generalized spike and wave pattern (fig. 14). This is the pattern that was classically

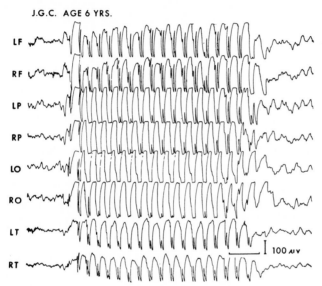

J.G.C. AGE 6 YRS.

LF
RF
LP
RP
LO
RO
LT
RT

I 100 µv

Figure 14. Paroxysmal seizure pattern of the classic 3 per second spike and wave type. This patient has had attacks of staring blankly for a few seconds since the age of 5 6/12 years. The child is considered to be very intelligent. There were no other abnormal findings.

associated with epilepsy and particularly with the so-called "petit mal." The implication of this pattern in a patient who has attacks of simple staring and unresponsiveness is that he has epilepsy of a particular type, namely, idiopathic. It should not be assumed, however, that the 3 per second spike and wave pattern is encountered only in patients who have lapse attacks. The pattern occurs almost as commonly in patients who have only generalized seizures. Thus, a history of generalized seizures plus the presence of 3 per second spike and wave pattern is diagnostic in the sense that the two add up to a form of epilepsy which is usually not associated with any demonstrable lesion of the brain and which has a significant familial incidence. It also provides definite differentiation of the clinical condition from epilepsy arising from symptomatic causes, such as the presence of a focal lesion of the brain or a diffuse encephalopathy of some type.

POLYSPIKE AND WAVE PATTERNS

It is believed by many that the paroxysmal spike and wave patterns in which the spike component predominates (that is, in which there are polyspike complexes or multiple spikes preceding the slow wave, such as are shown in figure 15) are more common

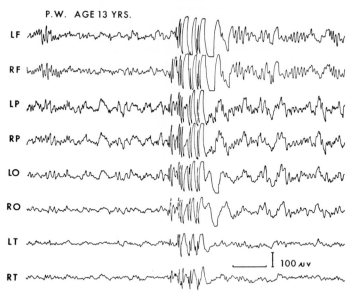

Figure 15.   Polyspike and wave bursts in sleep in a child who shows simple 3 per second spike and wave pattern awake. It is characteristic for this type of discharge to show more in sleep than in the waking record. This patient was referred because of a behavior problem at the age of 6. Simple absence type seizures had not been noticed until electroencephalographic findings (simple 3 per second spike and wave) brought them to the mother's attention. The onset of generalized seizures was at age 10.

in patients who have myoclonic jerks and/or generalized seizures. The presence of such abnormalities in a patient who has had only simple absence or lapse attacks thus may be considered reason for taking therapeutic steps toward protecting the patient from the onset of generalized seizures. For example, a patient with seizures of the absence type and a polyspike and wave pattern might be treated with a view to avoiding the possible activating effect that Tridione might have upon latent epilepsy (*i.e.*, by the addition of medication known to be effective against generalized seizures).

SLOW SPIKE AND WAVE PATTERNS

There are many forms of generalized spike and wave patterns, each having different implications in the evaluation of the patient. The classic pattern which has been described above and is associated with idiopathic epilepsy should be clearly differentiated from the generalized slow spike and wave types or variants, all of which are definitely a sign of a symptomatic or acquired disorder of the brain and have entirely different diagnostic and prognostic significance. There are several subgroups in this category, each having a different prognostic significance. Generally speaking, slow spike and wave patterns may be considered a sign of deteriorative change in neural elements. They are most commonly seen in children with clinical evidence of some degree of mental and motor impairment, and often the natural history is such as to suggest that they have arisen as a result of an insult to the brain which occurred as a result of a preceding inflammatory or other damaging process. Anoxic episodes and encephalitides, which are often unrecognized, are commonly the etiologic agents in the production of this type of abnormality. Thus, even in the absence of a clear-cut history suggesting cerebral insult, the presence of this sort of pattern in the electroencephalogram may be taken as evidence that some such insult has occurred. As an example, a thorough investigation of child L.L. was made because of the occurrence of generalized and akinetic seizures. The child showed some mild mental retardation and this was the only other abnormal finding. The electroencephalogram showed an almost continuous slow spike and wave dysrhythmia of the type illustrated in figure 16. In trying to find a reason for the electroencephalographic pattern, which is thought to be a sign of diffuse cerebral impairment, it was found that the mother had been exposed to rubella in the first trimester of pregnancy. Thus, by inference, it might be held that this patient suffered in utero an encephalitis which left him with a changed pattern of electrical activity and subsequent seizures, but without the other congenital abnormalities which are commonly associated with this type of early insult.

The most benign of these slow spike and wave patterns is the 2 per second "hump-wave" pattern, which occurs in paroxysms

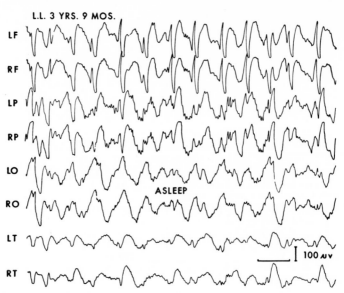

Figure 16. An almost continuous epileptiform activity of a slow, slow-spike and slow-wave type. There is little evidence of normal activity, and very little change in the electroencephalogram asleep or awake. At the age of 3 9/12 years the child began having attacks of sudden dropping to the floor, but got up immediately and apparently without change of consciousness (akinetic attacks). The child was premature two months and had a breech delivery. Development was quite slow; the child is clumsy and has incoordinated gait.

against a relatively normal background and a relatively normal alpha rhythm. The usual history of a patient showing this type of pattern is that, at about the age of 5 or 6 years, he suddenly developed attacks of falling accompanied by very brief, or not apparent, lapses of consciousness (so-called akinetic attacks). Also at about this time there was some decrease in the patient's mental efficiency, with an obvious setback in mental and motor development and an onset of behavior disorder. The seizures proved difficult to control, but the patient spontaneously ceased to have attacks after four or five years, and coincidentally the electroencephalographic evidence of the cerebral convulsive disorder markedly decreased or disappeared. In some cases, mental and motor impairment of some degree may persist.

As opposed to this more "benign" pattern, there are various electroencephalographic abnormalities of a similar character, such as the one shown in figure 17, in which the abnormality is more continuous, the background is more greatly disturbed and the alpha

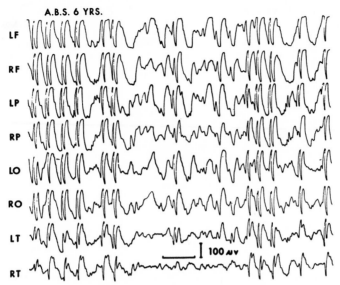

Figure 17. Generalized slow spike and wave dysrhythmia. The child was referred because of generalized tonic-clonic seizures and attacks of becoming limp and unresponsive with a blank stare but no muscular stiffness or jerking. These attacks began at the age of 5 years without evidence of preceding or inter-current illness. The child is moderately retarded mentally and has poor speech. There is history of a very difficult birth.

rhythm is either quite slow or entirely absent. In such cases, there is usually an earlier onset of seizures or mental retardation, or both. The prognosis is poorer in terms of continuing seizures, especially for spontaneous remission, and a moderate to marked degree of mental and motor retardation is the almost inevitable sequel.

A difference, which is of both clinical and theoretical signifi-cance, between the classic 3 per second spike and wave pattern and the slower patterns described above, is that the generalized spike and wave pattern of the classic type rarely occurs in the record for more than two or three seconds without the appearance of some ictal accompaniment, such as lapse of consciousness; on the other hand, the generalized slow patterns may be almost continuous in the record without a clinical sign of seizure activity.

HYPSARHYTHMIA

A dramatic pattern which is seen only in infants and young children consists of continuous high voltage activity of slow, sharp and polyspike type in all regions, with poor correlation between homologous areas on the two sides (fig. 18). Because of the extremely high voltage of the activity and its arrhythmic character, the abnormality has been called hypsarhythmia ("hypsi" meaning high).

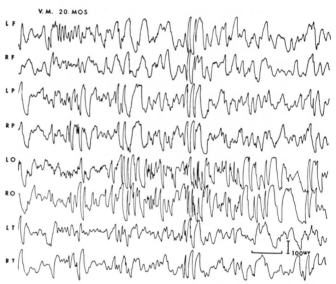

V. M. 20. MOS

LF
RF
LP
RP
LO
RO
LT
RT
100µv

Figure 18.   High voltage generalized slow, sharp and polyspike activity. The child has had attacks of sudden flexion of the neck and trunk (jackknife spells) since birth. These attacks sometimes occur in a short series of two to three in a group. The child is extremely hyperactive, and is unable to walk or talk now, at the age of 36 months.

Children showing this type of electrographic abnormality are generally subject to jackknife seizures or other similar attacks of the massive spasms group. Generalized tonic-clonic seizures also may occur in patients showing this pattern.

The prognosis is generally quite unfavorable insofar as mental and motor development is concerned, but occasional patients show remarkable recovery in later life. Seizures associated with this pattern are characteristically difficult to control, but sudden spontaneous remission is not uncommon.

The chief importance of this pattern is its prognostic significance, in that its presence in infancy might be the only objective evidence of brain damage at that early age.

14 AND 6 PER SECOND POSITIVE SPIKES

Recently, an electrographic pattern has been described which has a particular association with convulsive equivalent disorders. This pattern, an example of which is shown in figure 19, consists of a series of spikes repeating at a rate of 14 or 6 per second, located in the occipitotemporal region of the head but possibly

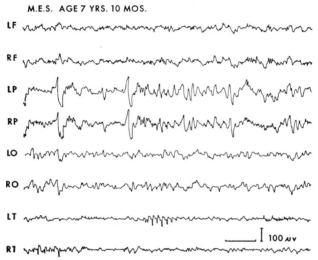

Figure 19.   Note bursts of 5 to 6 per second positive spikes in the left and right temporal leads in an otherwise normal sleep tracing. The patient was referred because of recurrent severe headaches over a period of three and one-half years.

taking origin in the hypothalamus or thalamus. This pattern is of great importance because it provides diagnostic information of the existence of epileptiform disorder in patients who have symptoms not often thought to be of this origin, and whose complaints are largely subjective.

It has been demonstrated that a relatively large number of children who have attacks of abdominal pain or headache, or both, with or without associated autonomic disturbances, such as flushing, pallor, nausea or vomiting, and in whom no visceral disease is evident, may have their attacks on the basis of epileptiform activity in the brain analogous to that which takes place when a convulsion occurs. The discharge in attacks, however, exclusively involves parts of the brain which have to do with visceral and sensory function.

That paroxysmal symptoms of a subjective type may originate in a brain disturbance akin to that of a convulsion and yet have no component suggesting a convulsion or even any alteration of consciousness, has been recognized for many years, but only recently has electrographic confirmation of this concept been forthcoming. The 14 and 6 per second positive spike pattern has a relatively specific correlation with this form of cerebral dysfunction. It should not be thought, however, that 14 and 6 per second positive spikes are seen only in patients with convulsive equivalent symptoms.

FOCAL ABNORMALITIES

It has been known for many years that localized lesions of the brain may cause focal discharges which may give rise to clinical seizures that can be either characteristic of the function of the part of the brain in which that lesion lies or be of the generalized tonic-clonic type. Early electroencephalographers demonstrated that in interseizure periods such localized lesions may give rise to focal abnormal discharge arising in the area involved. This discharge may be continuous or sporadic, and vary considerably in wave form and voltage. It may consist of random spikes or of sharp waves or slow spikes, or even of slow waves. Uncommonly, the discharge may consist of fast activity arising locally from a circumscribed area. Originally, it was thought that epileptogenic lesions—that is, lesions that give rise to seizures—are always characterized by spike discharge, but this has since been proved not to be so. At the time of a seizure, spikes are generally produced, but in the interseizure period the focal discharge may show wave forms of any one of, or a mixture of, any of the above. The importance of discovering a focal discharging abnormality in the electroencephalogram lies in the fact that such foci, although circumscribed and localized to a given place, may give rise to symptoms which clinically have no localizing signs. Thus, it is not uncommon for a discharging epileptogenic lesion, for example, in the temporal lobe, to give rise only to generalized seizures without any clinical evidence of local onset.

Once it is proved that the seizure arises focally, that is, from a focal point in the brain, it must be assumed that there is an underlying localized lesion of the brain producing this discharge. It then becomes necessary to determine the nature of that lesion—whether it is an expanding lesion or a static lesion, such as a scar or microgyrus.

The electroencephalogram may be helpful in arriving at this differentiation, but in most patients, especially in adults, other procedures such as pneumoencephalography may be required. However, a discussion of the diagnostic usefulness of electroencephalography would be incomplete without pointing out that in children the sporadic localized slow-spike discharge of the type illustrated in figure 20 is diagnostic of a focal atrophic lesion, or, at least, of a focal *non-*

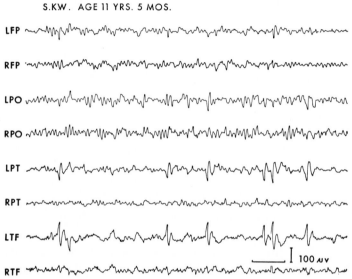

S.KW. AGE 11 YRS. 5 MOS.

Figure 20. Repeated slow-spike discharges in the region of the left temporal electrode. The record otherwise is fairly normal. The patient was referred for attacks of suddenly becoming unable to speak, with his tongue feeling numb followed by a slight twitching of the right corner of his mouth. A neurological examination showed no abnormality.

neoplastic lesion, and that it is therefore not necessary to resort to more drastic procedures in the fear that such patients might have brain tumors. (Other types of focal spike activity may be associated with a neoplasm and the correlation refers only to the particular pattern described above.)

MULTIFOCAL ABNORMALITIES

Electrograms showing several independent foci of spike discharge (fig. 21) are not uncommon in children. Apparently they are evidence of the existence in the brain of multiple cortical atrophic

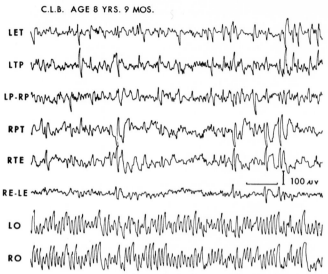

C.L.B. AGE 8 YRS. 9 MOS.

LET

LTP

LP-RP

RPT

RTE

RE-LE

100 µv

LO

RO

Figure 21. Multiple independent foci of spike discharge in the left temporal, right temporal and left and right parietal regions. The background activity is also abnormal, the waking record being too slow. The patient has had generalized seizures and several types of focal motor seizures with variable onset and characteristics; this often occurs in patients with multifocal records. The child is mentally retarded and is subject to numerous unprovoked episodes of aggressive and destructive behavior.

areas which are the source of discharge that is potentially epilepto-genic. Children with this type of electroencephalogram may show several varying types of seizure, *e.g.*, focal motor, sensory and ad-versive seizures may occur at different times in the same patient. The prognosis is generally not good for motor and mental develop-ment and there is often evidence of neurological abnormality, especially when the background activity is also quite abnormal.

Whether the record shows a unifocal or multifocal abnormality, the prognosis is much affected by the character of the background activity. Thus, the prognosis is much poorer in the case of a single focus when, in addition, there is evidence of diffuse abnormality, especially if it is of the fast type shown in figure 22.

5 TO 6 PER SECOND SPIKE AND WAVE (SPIKE AND WAVE PHANTOM)

There are several patterns which are relatively rare but which, nevertheless, have a high, diagnostically correlative value. The most common of these is the 5 to 6 per second spike and wave pattern of

E.R.D. AGE 3 YRS.

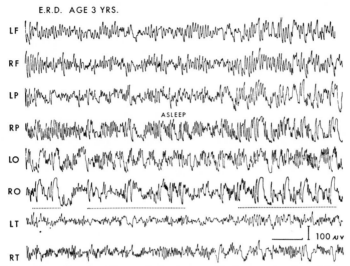

Figure 22.   Focal spike and slow-wave discharges in the right occipital region (underlined). There is continuous high voltage fast activity and spindling in all areas. The patient has spastic cerebral palsy, the left side being more affected. He has focal motor seizures beginning in the left face and arm without loss of consciousness. He is moderately retarded, and has very poor vision, especially in the left eye.

low voltage known as the *spike-wave phantom.* This is an epileptiform finding more commonly seen in adults than children and its importance lies in the fact that it is often found in older patients presenting with a first seizure; its presence points to a convulsive disorder and rules against the obvious possibility of neoplasm. It is mostly seen in patients with a history of attacks that resemble faints, but generalized seizures are also common.

PAROXYSMAL BILATERAL SLOW BURSTS

Paroxysmal bilateral slow activity in the waking records of either adults or children is generally considered an epileptiform finding. The definition of what constitutes *paroxysmal* is sometimes not clear in the young child, and this is a possible source of error. However, any activity occurring in a burst in the fully awake adult, that is, where there is a sudden and marked increase in voltage, with or without a change in frequency, may be considered to be of this kind. Paroxysmal generalized patterns are nonspecific in terms of particular clinical entities, but they are considered to suggest dysfunction at a deep midline (thalamic?) level. They occur in various conditions and may be seen, for example, as a residual of head injury and encephalitis, and may, in fact, occur in idiopathic epilepsy. They are nondiagnostic both in terms of the underlying abnormality and of etiology.

SIMPLE DYSRHYTHMIA

The classically normal adult electroencephalogram consists of a simple, well regulated, sinusoidal rhythm of from 8 to 12 per second which arises in the occipital region bilaterally, and a low voltage fast activity in anterior head regions. There is, however, considerable variation in this pattern among normal adults; in a small percentage of normal adults activity is present which is slower than 8 and in others much more fast activity is present than characterizes the classically normal record as described above. Records in which there is simply more fast activity or higher voltage fast activity, or more slow activity than normal, are called "dysrhythmic." Thus, a simple "fast" dysrhythmia merely means a record in which there is an excess of fast activity or higher voltage fast activity than is normally encountered. A "slow" dysrhythmia merely refers to one in which there is more slow activity present than normal or in which the alpha rhythm is slower than normal for age. When sampling of an epileptic and a normal population is made, it is found that the incidence of simple dysrhythmias is far greater in the epileptic than in the normal population. For this reason, the presence of dysrhythmia in a patient suspected of having an epileptic disorder might be considered "supportive" evidence for a clinical diagnosis of epilepsy. However, such findings are quite nonspecific and occur in many conditions in which convulsive symptoms are not present. Indeed, they may occur in mild form as an idiosyncrasy in people with no apparent neurological disease. The degree of dysrhythmia present is, of course, the important factor in evaluating its significance with regard to a patient's history and findings; thus, the more pronounced the abnormality, the more likely it is that a reliable correlation can be made.

Prognostic Uses of Electroencephalography

The prognostic evaluation of the patient with an epileptic disorder may be greatly helped by the electroencephalographic findings at the time that the original diagnosis is made and throughout the course of therapy and management. This help may be derived in two ways: (1) in predicting the course of the disease, and (2) as a guide in regulating the patient's therapeutic regimen.

PREDICTION OF THE COURSE OF THE DISEASE

The original electrographic findings have prognostic significance in terms of the outcome for the patient in relation to the number of seizures, in the ease with which such seizures may be controlled, and in the evaluation and differentiation of nonprogressive from progressive pathology. In children, the possibility of predicting future mental and motor development will be greatly influenced by the original and subsequent electrographic findings. The following may be considered reliable factors of prognostic evaluation in these terms:

(1) A normal electroencephalogram in the patient, whether child or adult, with known convulsions or epileptic symptoms may be considered a good prognostic sign, in that, statistically, patients presenting with normal electroencephalograms show less in the way of neurological deficit, generally show a better response to medication, and rarely show progressive deterioration or deficit.

(2) Demonstration of the classic 3 per second spike and wave pattern against a normal background in a patient with the classic absence seizures may be considered a good prognostic sign, in that such findings rule against the presence of palpable cerebral pathology. The outlook for mental and motor development is generally good. While the control of seizures may be difficult initially, there is a strong chance for spontaneous remission as the child reaches his teens or early adulthood.

(3) Demonstration of slow-spike and wave diffuse patterns is a prognostically poorer sign, both in terms of control of seizures and in terms of motor and mental development. Some degree of variation is interpretable even within this group; thus, the pattern shown in figure 16 is a poorer prognostic finding than is the pattern shown in figure 17 (pp. 104, 105).

(4) If interpretation and evaluation are based largely upon the natural history of such cases, the 14 and 6 per second positive spike pattern may be considered to have a relatively good prognostic significance. It has been demonstrated that, although such patients are sometimes refractory to drug therapy and require considerable

experimentation in order to find an effective agent for the control of attacks, if this is their sole electrographic abnormality they usually do not have evidence of other neurological abnormality and do not develop any. When this pattern is present in children, both the pattern and the clinical symptoms generally will disappear before adolescence or in the adolescent period.

(5) In infants and young children, the demonstration of hypsa-rhythmia is a poor prognostic feature in that it is almost inevitable that there will be some degree of mental and motor retardation; however, the spontaneous remission of seizures in later childhood is not uncommon in this group.

(6) Circumscribed focal abnormalities in otherwise normal elec-troencephalograms have a better prognostic significance than all other forms of electroencephalographic abnormalities, with the exception of 14 and 6 per second positive spikes and the classic 3 per second spike and wave pattern. Indeed, in children, the demonstration of a focal slow-spike abnormality in the midtemporal region may consti-tute the most benign, in terms of its natural history, of any sympto-matic finding known (fig. 20). In these children, the seizures are generally easy to control, and the abnormality and seizures usually disappear in late childhood or early adulthood; the incidence of temporary or persisting neurological deficit is relatively low.

(7) Focal abnormality existing against a background which is diffusely abnormal is a poorer prognostic finding than the purely focal record and is often a sign of both diffuse and focal involvement of the brain (fig. 22). However, it is possible in certain instances for the focal discharge to disrupt the total activity of the brain so that when and if the focal discharge is curbed through the use of surgery or medication the generalized disturbance will subside, thus indicating that the essential abnormality was primarily focal.

(8) Paroxysmal slow activity against a normal background may be a relatively good prognostic electrographic finding; however, this evaluation is much less assured than that given above for the other types of abnormality.

Perhaps the greatest error of electrographic evaluation is the one of trying to equate the dramatic character of an electrographic abnormality with the severity of the patient's symptoms. Thus, a monorhythmic dysrhythmia—by which we mean, for example, an electroencephalogram consisting of little except low voltage 5 to 6 per second rhythmic waves such as those shown in figure 23—may have a much greater significance in terms of clinical abnormality and underlying pathology than does a record in which there is a dramatic demonstration of numerous high voltage 3 per second spike

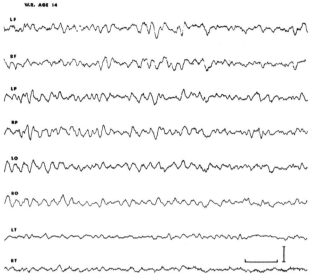

Figure 23.   Almost continuous 5 to 6 per second rhythmic activity in all leads. There is little evidence of any other type of activity in the entire recording. The patient was normal until about 5 years, at which time he began to show personality changes and developed generalized seizures. There was progressive mental and motor retardation from then on. Histologic diagnosis: cerebral lipoidosis.

and wave bursts. This is because such a finding may be a sign of deterioration and, therefore, in spite of its undramatic character, a sign of a diffuse encephalopathy of severe degree. Thus, it is almost impossible to equate the degree of (nonspecific) dysrhythmia as such with the severity of the epilepsy or even of an underlying encephalopathy.

ELECTROENCEPHALOGRAPHY IN REGULATION OF THE THERAPEUTIC REGIMEN

When reduction or stoppage of medication is contemplated, it is usually desirable to make a follow-up electrographic study; however, the evaluation of the findings must be carried out with the following in mind:

(1) Absence of electroencephalographic abnormality cannot be

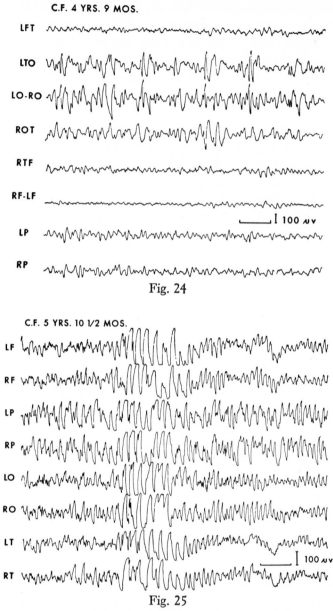

Fig. 24

Fig. 25

Figures 24 and 25. The first of these two electroencephalograms (fig. 24) was made when the patient was first seen at a time when he was having many seizures. The second sample (fig. 25) is taken from a record made when the patient had been seizure-free for one year. The second tracing showed paroxysmal generalized bursts (as shown above) in addition to the spike focus (not shown).

considered definite guarantee that the patient will not have seizures if medication is reduced or discontinued. Nevertheless, the demonstration of a normal electroencephalogram both awake and asleep and during overventilation may be considered good support for a clinical decision to reduce or discontinue medication.

(2) Persistence of electroencephalographic abnormality and even, to some degree, a worsening of the electroencephalographic findings (figs. 24 and 25) cannot be considered definite evidence that the patient needs to be continued on medication. This decision must, in many cases, be made solely on clinical grounds because it has been demonstrated repeatedly that many patients, who clinically cease to have seizures and remain seizure-free for months and even years when taken off medication, may continue to be free of seizures in spite of the electroencephalogram continuing to be grossly abnormal and having essentially the same character as the premedication record.

(3) The effect of the medication itself must be borne in mind in evaluating the abnormality of the electroencephalogram following drug treatment. It has been shown, for example, that the barbiturates, Mesantoin, and, to a lesser degree, meprobamate, chlorpromazine and similar drugs, produce fast activity in the electroencephalogram which may be quite pronounced. Also such drugs in large amounts may increase slow activity or produce slow activity where it was not present before.

The question as to whether or not anticonvulsant drugs reduce seizures by abolishing the abnormal activity of the brain is a complicated one which has a different answer for each of the drugs involved; to a larger extent, it is influenced by the type of electroencephalographic abnormality and the clinical pathological condition. It is known that Tridione, when it is effective in controlling idiopathic seizures, often will reduce or abolish 3 per second spike and wave activity in the electroencephalogram. On the whole, though, it can be said that most drugs exert their effect in controlling seizures without necessarily reducing the degree of abnormality in the electroencephalogram or altering its character. Thus, it should not be considered that a drug has been ineffective if clinical control is obtained, yet the electroencephalographic abnormality remains unchanged, because, in most cases, this is all that can be expected of the drugs presently available.

CHAPTER 15

Management of Seizures

Sᴵɴᴄᴇ EPILEPSY is merely a symptom and occasionally a sign of disturbed cerebral function, the clinician must first decide whether the seizures are symptomatic or idiopathic or merely a reflection of primary extracerebral disorder. If the epilepsy is thought to be symptomatic, the clinician must determine whether the pathological process is focal or diffuse and whether it is progressive or static.

The character of the seizure may indicate that the causative lesion is a focal one and point to its localization. But, while a focal onset to a seizure favors a focal lesion, a generalized seizure without focal signs does not exclude the possibility that the underlying pathology is focal, since focal cerebral lesions often produce seizures which have no localizing features.

The presence of abnormal neurological signs strengthens the possibility of an underlying cerebral lesion, but the absence of abnormal findings on neurological examination does not exclude such a diagnosis. Discrete focal lesions may be evident only in the seizures they produce.

The age of onset and the length of time that the patient has been having seizures are helpful in deciding whether an epileptogenic lesion is expanding or atrophic. An early age of onset and

119

many years of seizures favor the diagnosis of an atrophic lesion. If an atrophic lesion, such as a microgyrus or a cerebral scar, is the cause of seizures, the history may provide evidence as to its cause. A history of a severe birth injury or of trauma to the head may provide the clue to etiology. Inflammatory brain disease, in spite of being diffuse, as in meningoencephalitis, may cause focal epileptogenic lesions. If the physical examination reveals a facial nevus or multiple congenital anomalies, then epilepsy is more likely to be on the basis of an associated malformation of the brain.

If the clinical picture and investigation by roentgenogram, electroencephalography, angiography or air encephalography reveal evidence of an expanding lesion, the type of lesion must be determined and the desirability of its removal considered. After the excision of a brain tumor, a cerebral abscess or other space-occupying lesion, seizures may cease and anticonvulsant medication may be withdrawn gradually. However, seizures may persist after surgery and require continued medication.

Medical control of seizures involves the use of proper anticonvulsant drugs, psychological measures to improve the mental state of the patient and maintenance of general good health.

Medication

The control of seizures usually depends more upon proper medication than on any other single factor. Choice of medication depends on the seizure pattern, the type of electroencephalographic abnormality, the side effects of the drugs and, to a lesser degree, the cost of the drugs. The type of attack is the most important single consideration in determining the choice of medication.

GENERALIZED SEIZURES

Generalized seizures are usually the most easily controlled of all seizure types. They respond best, as a rule, to the hydantoinates, particularly Dilantin, but the barbiturate anticonvulsants, such as phenobarbital and Mebaral, are often quite effective. Mysoline is also an effective drug in the control of generalized seizures.

Dilantin is generally considered to have the greatest scope of usefulness of all the anticonvulsants. It has some effectiveness in all but lapse and akinetic seizures and at the same time a low incidence of noxious side effects. It has a wide margin of safety with regard to toxicity, and large doses (up to 5 gm.) have been taken without serious consequence. Occasional patients, because of idiosyncrasies, cannot tolerate even small doses of this drug. Such cases may have severe vomiting and irritability (infants) with small doses of Dilantin. Other effects include skin rash, fever and, very rarely, hepatitis and bone marrow depression. Undesirable side effects of Dilantin are gum hypertrophy and occasionally hirsutism.

Signs of overdosage which are commonly encountered are ataxia, nystagmus, diplopia, lassitude and constipation.

Gum hypertrophy is common and is not an indication for stopping the drug. The patient should be instructed to massage his gums each time he brushes his teeth, because this inhibits excessive swelling. Vitamin C may be useful if bleeding of the gums occurs. If unsteadiness or double vision develops, the drug should be decreased or discontinued for a few days (increasing other medication in order to avoid status epilepticus), and then restarted at a lower dosage. The occurrence of skin rash calls for immediate discontinuation of the medication; when the rash has faded, the drug may cautiously be tried again, to be discontinued permanently if the rash reappears. Nausea and vomiting, which occur chiefly in infants, is another cause for discontinuation of the drug. Depression of the bone marrow and hepatic damage are so rare that they should not discourage the general use of Dilantin. It is not necessary to do periodic blood examinations in patients receiving Dilantin. Dilantin rarely produces drowsiness, and this lack of soporific effect is one of its main advantages.

The usual procedure is to begin with a moderate dosage, appropriate to the age and weight of the patient (Drug Table, p. 138), and to increase the amount of medication if the seizures are not controlled within a week or 10 days. If the seizures continue to be frequent with the maximal doses of Dilantin tolerated by the patient, then a barbiturate should be added in supplemental doses.

Phenobarbital is the most effective and inexpensive barbiturate for adults and older children. However, it may produce excessive irritability in infants and younger children. For this reason, Mebaral is often used instead of phenobarbital in these younger patients. The dosages of phenobarbital and Mebaral are shown in the Drug

Table. Dilantin and phenobarbital when combined constitute the most generally effective combination for the control of focal and generalized convulsions. Phenobarbital or Mebaral alone may be quite effective in the treatment of generalized convulsions.

The side effects of these drugs include drowsiness, dullness, unsteadiness, skin rash and irritability. Drowsiness and dullness constitute an indication for reduction in the dosage of phenobarbital and the addition of some other anticonvulsant. Ataxia is also a reason for reduction in dosage. Skin rashes may occur, and according to the severity of the rash the dosage may be reduced or the drug discontinued. If these medicines are suddenly stopped, the patient should be protected against status epilepticus by other agents having a lesser tendency to produce skin rashes (paraldehyde). When the rash has cleared, the drug may cautiously be restarted. The rash may then not return, but if it does, the drug should not be given any more. If Dilantin and phenobarbital or Dilantin and Mebaral are not effective in controlling seizures, other medications may be added or substituted.

Mesantoin may be effective where Dilantin fails. This drug is more likely, however, to produce skin rashes and depression of bone marrow than Dilantin; thus, white and differential blood counts and hemoglobin determinations should be done at monthly intervals for a year after medication is begun and less frequently later. Mesantoin very rarely produces gum hypertrophy.

Mysoline is another effective drug which may be tried if Dilantin and phenobarbital prove ineffective. It may be combined with Dilantin but is usually too soporific when given with the barbiturates. The dosage of Mysoline must be built up gradually over six to eight days in order to avoid the marked drowsiness and ataxia which appear if the drug is begun in full dosage immediately. The dosage is indicated in the Drug Table. Other less common side effects of Mysoline are skin rashes and leukopenia.

Celontin is a fairly potent anticonvulsant, recently introduced. It has proved quite helpful in generalized and temporal lobe seizures. It also has proved useful in the control of akinetic and myoclonic seizures of symptomatic origin and occasionally has reduced attacks of the massive spasm type. High doses may produce unsteadiness.

Gemonil is a barbiturate with anticonvulsant action which has the advantages of low toxicity and few side effects. Its greatest usefulness is in the treatment of massive spasms.

FOCAL SEIZURES

Focal seizures, whether manifest in motor or sensory spheres, are treated along the same lines as indicated in the treatment of generalized convulsions. Thus, the hydantoinates and barbiturates, as well as Mysoline and Celontin, may be effective here.

Psychomotor attacks, when they are manifestations of discharging temporal lobe lesions, are often more difficult to control than generalized or other varieties of focal seizures. Dilantin is often effective; Mesantoin also may be helpful. Celontin is probably the next most useful of the anticonvulsants in the treatment of this type of seizure. The addition of Mysoline or occasionally phenobarbital to Dilantin or Mesantoin may be a further help.

Phenurone is a drug which occasionally proves effective in psychomotor epilepsy. Although it is a powerful anticonvulsant, its usefulness is limited by frequent and dangerous toxic side effects. It is hepatotoxic and often produces leukopenia. It may lead to irritability in the young and to a toxic psychosis in older patients. Phenurone should be used only when other agents prove ineffective. Monthly blood counts and urinary urobilinogen determinations are mandatory.

MASSIVE SPASMS

It is very difficult and often impossible to completely suppress attacks of the massive spasm type. In our hands a combination of Gemonil and Mebaral has proved to be the most effective treatment. Other drugs (meprobamate, Celontin, Dilantin, phenobarbital, Phenurone and Milontin) may be tried if this combination does not prove helpful. More recently ACTH or cortisone has been reported to be effective in the treatment of massive spasms.

LAPSE OR ABSENCE ATTACKS

The most effective drug in the treatment of lapse attacks (petit mal absence) is Tridione. It has been reported that this drug may precipitate generalized seizures in patients who have not had such attacks previously, but it is difficult to say whether or not these patients would have developed convulsions anyway. Experience has shown that the possibility of precipitating generalized seizures in the patient with idiopathic lapse attacks by using Tridione alone is negligible. However, the electroencephalographic findings may justifiably influence the physician to use phenobarbital, or a similar drug, in combination with Tridione if polyspike, or paroxysmal, or high voltage fast bursts are present. Where lapse and generalized attacks both occur in the same patient, Tridione is best combined with Dilantin or phenobarbital.

Tridione has only slight soporific effects. Skin rashes are not uncommon, but the major toxic effect of Tridione is on the blood-forming elements, and serious, even fatal, depression of bone marrow has followed its use. This necessitates regular monthly white and differential blood counts in patients receiving Tridione. If the total polymorphonuclear count drops below 2,000 per cubic millimeter, the dosage should be decreased or the drug stopped. Weekly blood counts should be done if the number of white cells is depressed or if the patient develops an infection. Photophobia, hiccups, eosinophilia and nephrosis are other less common toxic effects. Fear of possible toxic effects of Tridione has led physicians to use it in doses which are too small to be effective. With careful watching of the patient, relatively large doses can be safely used (Drug Table).

Paradione may be tried if a patient reacts adversely to Tridione. It is less toxic but also much less effective than Tridione.

Milontin is sometimes effective against lapse attacks but is more useful in combination with Tridione. Milontin occasionally produces hematuria and albuminuria but is relatively nontoxic.

Diamox is second in effectiveness to Tridione in the control of lapse attacks. It is particularly effective in patients showing marked activation by overventilation. The commonest side effect is anorexia with resultant weight loss. Occasionally, children complain of drowsiness when taking Diamox. Paresthesias also sometimes occur but are rare. The drug is expensive and the cost may limit its use.

Meprobamate (Equanil, Miltown) has some anticonvulsant activity in addition to its tranquilizing effect. It is moderately effective in lapse attacks, and the only side effect of note is drowsiness at high dosage levels.

The amphetamines (Dexedrine and Benzedrine) are occasionally helpful in absence attacks, but they are of limited usefulness and may produce hyperirritability, sleeplessness and loss of appetite.

Antimalarials, especially chloroquine, have recently been reported effective in lapse attacks.

MYOCLONIC ATTACKS

The myoclonic seizures which occur in idiopathic epilepsy usually show good response to the same drugs which are effective in the treatment of lapse attacks. Celontin has proved effective in the control of myoclonic attacks of symptomatic origin.

AKINETIC ATTACKS

Akinetic attacks, or their partial expression, head-nodding spells, usually are quite resistant to drug therapy. The medications noted above as useful in lapse and myoclonic attacks may be tried. Gemonil or other barbiturates may also be helpful.

CONVULSIVE EQUIVALENT (AUTONOMIC, PAIN AND RAGE) ATTACKS

Most "equivalent" attacks respond to Dilantin, Mesantoin or barbiturates, or a combination of these drugs. When, however, these attacks are resistant to these medications, Diamox, meprobamate or Tridione may be effective.

STATUS EPILEPTICUS

Occasionally, generalized seizures occur so rapidly, one after another, that the patient does not recover consciousness between attacks. This is called "epileptic status." It may occur when a medication is abruptly discontinued or changed. Epileptic status is a medical emergency, for if the attacks are not soon stopped there is a considerable (10 per cent) mortality.

The immediate aim of treatment is to stop the seizures and to prevent recurrence. Intravenous paraldehyde, given slowly, is a most effective measure. Intravenous Nembutal or Sodium Amytal is also useful in controlling the immediate convulsions. The essence of success in the treatment of status is not so much the control of the immediate seizure, for any central nervous system depressant may accomplish this, but the prevention of recurrent seizures. To this end phenobarbital given intramuscularly or Dilantin given intravenously may be given in repeated doses until the patient can take oral medication. As soon as the patient regains consciousness, he should be given combined Dilantin and phenobarbital medication by mouth. Paraldehyde given by stomach tube or rectally may be employed for a day or two as supportive therapy. If the status is due to discontinuation of medication, this medication should, if possible, be given again. The administration of oxygen to patients in status helps to reduce cerebral anoxemia and thus to control the status, as well as prevent brain injury due to anoxia.

Anesthesia with ether or Avertin has been employed by some for the control of very refractory cases of status epilepticus; however, it is doubtful whether this is really very effective, and such drawbacks as respiratory depression or pulmonary congestion outweigh its possible benefit.

Patients in status epilepticus are liable to aspirate saliva or vomitus, and it is useful to give penicillin prophylactically to prevent pneumonia. Maintenance of a free airway, removal of secretions, regular repositioning and maintenance of fluid balance and nutrition are all essential features of the proper management of status.

Repeated seizures without intermission may occur with other types of attack, particularly focal motor (epilepsia partialis continua), psychomotor and absence attacks. The treatment of focal motor and psychomotor status is essentially the same as for generalized status epilepticus. When lapse attacks of idiopathic epilepsy become almost continuous, it is often difficult to return the patient to a normal state of consciousness, and various approaches to the problem may have to be tried before an effective measure is found. Large doses of Tridione or intravenous Diamox or both may be effective, but if the status persists, it may be necessary to resort to starvation followed by a ketogenic diet.

Other Drugs

Paraldehyde is one of the safest drugs useful in epilepsy. Its main place is in the treatment of status epilepticus, but it is also used in protecting patients from possible seizures when it becomes necessary to stop Dilantin or other drugs quickly as a result of a serious adverse reaction. The main objection to paraldehyde is its unpleasant odor and taste. If given intramuscularly, it may cause the development of a sterile abscess. Slow intravenous administration is often helpful in arresting status. It may be given undiluted, slowly, intravenously or diluted in isotonic solution (see the Drug Table, for dosage). Intravenous administration should be stopped as soon as the seizure ends. The unpleasant odor precludes the use of paraldehyde as a long-term medication.

Bromides were early used in the treatment of seizures and are still being used by some mail-order drug dispensing agencies. They have anticonvulsant properties but usually produce marked drowsiness in effective doses. The concentration of the bromide ion in the blood is the significant factor in the action of the drug, irrespective of the particular salt used. Toxic effects include an acneiform rash, mental agitation and tremulousness. Bromides are seldom indicated in present-day practice.

Ketogenic Diet

If an effective drug is not found or if effective medication must be discontinued because of drug idiosyncrasy, the ketogenic diet may be tried as a last resort. This diet may prove helpful in children under 9 years of age. The intelligent cooperation of the patient's parents is essential because of the difficulties in having the child maintain the unappetizing high fat and low carbohydrate regime. The diet is initiated by a three to four day period of starvation; the high fat diet is then begun. Fats make up about 80 per cent by weight of the diet. An adequate level of ketosis is indicated by persistent ketonuria.

Management of Psychological Problems

The epileptic patient has to contend with special social, psychological and, if an adult, economic problems. The epileptic child may be barred from school because of unfounded fear or ignorance. The patient and his family may be shunned by their neighbors because of belief that the condition is associated with insanity and is a sign of an hereditary stigma, because of superstition concerning the supernatural cause of seizures or because of suspicion that the condition is infectious. Education of the public is improving the lot of seizure patients, but much misinformation persists.

Embarrassment caused by convulsions or by bizarre behavior in psychomotor attacks in public places may lead the patient to withdraw from society. The family of an epileptic may reject him or may try to hide his condition from their friends. On the other hand, the patient's family may become overprotective and in this way interfere with the patient's activities and potential development. An adult epileptic may lose his job because of seizures, and this adds economic stress to an already troublesome problem. Frustration by excessive inhibition produces tension which is psychologically harmful and which may, in turn, precipitate more seizures.

Explanation to the patient and his relatives that seizures may be a result of a scar in the brain or of a greater than usual excitability of the brain usually relieves much of the anxiety associated with epilepsy. Encouragement to lead an active life often gives the well controlled seizure patient an opportunity to attend school or take a job, giving him a feeling of satisfaction and accomplishment.

The doctor's explanation of the role of medication in controlling the seizures and the necessity for adherence to a regular dosage schedule is a very important factor in the control of the patient's seizures. If the patient understands the importance of medication and the need to take it regularly, he is far more likely to take it faithfully. The expected duration of treatment should also be discussed as soon as a diagnosis is made.

Certain limitations of activity are necessary in epileptic individuals. The frequency and character of the patient's seizures will determine the feasibility of such potentially dangerous activities as riding a bicycle or driving a car. Similarly, a patient with seizures should not be permitted to swim unaccompanied or beyond his depth or to climb to heights from which a fall would endanger his life or limbs. He should not be allowed to work with or near exposed machinery or in areas close to other hazards into which he might fall. Certainly, a seizure patient should not drive an automobile until he has been free of seizures for two years, for an attack while driving would endanger not only his life but other lives as well. Generally, with the exception of the foregoing limitations, a patient with seizures should be encouraged to live as normal and full a life as possible.

Genetic Problems

The occurrence of epileptic seizures in a member of a family often causes anxiety to the family because of fears concerning the possible role of genetic or congenital factors in the disorder. A couple with an only child who has seizures may wonder if any other children they might have would be similarly afflicted. In all but a relatively few cases, reassurance that this is unlikely can be given. If the seizures are symptomatic, the role of genetic factors will be minor or nonexistent and, even if idiopathic, will not be of great significance unless both parents have a positive family history of seizures. The statistics are not entirely reliable because of the difficulty of obtaining a comprehensive and dependable family history. If only one parent is epileptic, the chances of any offspring being epileptic are about 1 in 40. If both have a history of chronic seizures, the chances are still only 1 in 4.

This data can also serve as reassurance to the epileptic himself in terms of the advisability of his marrying and having children. However, if the cause of the epilepsy is one of the heredofamilial diseases, such as lipoidosis or phenylketonuria, the outlook is, of course, the reverse, and transmission of the disease and of the secondary seizures is very likely.

Probably one of the most important factors with which the physician has to deal in the care of epileptics is the guilt felt by a parent or parents over their imagined responsibility for their child having seizures. At various times, alcoholism, syphilis and masturbation have been implicated as the cause of seizures in the offspring of the offender. Anxiety concerning these or even more vaguely realized self implications as the cause of a child's seizures must often be dispelled by careful explanation of the nature of the disorder and of the rarity of parental culpability in its genesis.

Surgery in Epilepsy

Neurosurgical measures may be helpful where a focal abnormality of the brain is the cause of seizures. If the lesion does not in itself require extirpation, therapy can be directed entirely toward control of the seizures by medical means. If, on the other hand, the lesion is progressive, it is this factor and not the seizures which is of prime importance in determining if surgery is to be carried out. The indication for surgery in these instances is determined by the character of the lesion and not by the seizure state. In patients with atrophic epileptogenic lesions, surgery is only indicated when medical control fails.

Several prerequisites must be met before consideration should be given to surgical intervention in cases in which the lesion is a cortical scar or microgyrus. The first of these is that a thorough effort to obtain medical control has failed. By failure is meant no control or poor control of incapacitating seizures after an exhaustive trial of the various anticonvulsant drugs in adequate dosage, alone or in combination, over a period of at least a year. The second prerequisite is the determination that the seizures do originate in a circumscribed part of the brain, the excision of which would not be unduly disabling. The probability that surgical excision will relieve the patient of seizures or will significantly reduce the seizure frequency is determined by numerous factors, such as the extent of cerebral damage. However, with proper patient selection and with experience, corticectomy has resulted in a cessation of attacks in 40 per cent and in improvement in a further 35 per cent of patients undergoing surgery.

There are many considerations which limit the applicability of surgical excision of epileptogenic cortical scars. A mortality rate of about 1.5 per cent, even in experienced hands, is an important one. The possibility of a greater functional deficit after surgery is a further consideration. Excision of the cerebral cortex in the motor region and in those parts of the brain concerned with speech may be followed by hemiparesis or aphasic disturbances which are as troublesome or more so than the original seizures. Economic considerations, such as the expense of necessary investigation and surgical therapy, may also prove limiting factors.

The location and extent of surgical removal are governed by the preoperative evidence of localization as provided by the seizure pattern, the electroencephalogram and air studies. At craniotomy, the appearance of the cortex and the findings of electrocorticography further influence the excision. In general, surgical removal is limited largely to the abnormally discharging cortex.

In patients with seizures and behavior disorder who also have evidence of gross unilateral brain damage, in particular hemiplegia and hemianopia, removal of the entire damaged hemisphere (hemispherectomy) may be of value. The procedure can be carried out in such patients without producing further neurological deficit and has proved effective in the control of seizures and behavior disorder.

EXAMPLE: *Surgery*

J.W., Clinic No. B-155

At 9 days of age this patient began to have seizures. Her head drew back, her limbs jerked and she became cyanotic. One seizure on the ninth day of life lasted for five to six hours. She continued to have several generalized seizures daily, in spite of medication with Dilantin and phenobarbital.

At 18 months of age the child suddenly developed a right hemiplegia, which cleared over the next few days. At 4 6/12 years a right hemiplegia suddenly recurred. The paralysis gradually lessened over a period of a few weeks, but after this she had persistent weakness of the right hand and stiffness of the right lower limb.

The seizures stopped spontaneously at 7 years, but at 11 years of age they recurred. The patient became fretful and groaned a few minutes before an attack. Her head and eyes pulled to the right and then generalized jerking developed. Some of the convulsions involved the right side only. She was admitted to the Blue Bird Clinic, and Dilantin, Mebaral, phenobarbital and Tridione were given in unsuccessful attempts to control her seizures.

Her birth weight had been 5 1/2 lbs.; jaundice developed the first day and persisted for four weeks. Her development was slow; she sat unsupported at 1 year, walked at 2 years and spoke single words clearly at 3 years. She did fairly well in school except for poor arithmetic grades. There was no history of neurological disorder in the family.

An examination when the patient was 11 years revealed a right spastic hemiparesis with right-sided hemiatrophy. The myotatic reflexes were hyperactive on the right.

The EEG showed a grossly disordered record with continuous focal epileptiform activity arising in the left superior central region. Angiography and pneumoencephalography were performed and showed no abnormality. In view of persistent seizures occurring several times daily, surgical removal of the epileptogenic focus was attempted using electrocorticographic localization. However, the child continued to have several seizures daily in which her mouth pulled to the right and her right limbs jerked for about a minute. Various drugs, including Dilantin, Mebaral, Mysoline, Mesantoin and paraldehyde, were used in various combinations in fruitless efforts to stop the attacks. Because a supplementary motor focus was suggested by the development of attacks characterized by a turning of the head and eyes to the right, facing the open palm of the uplifted right hand, depth electrodes were placed in the mesial aspect of the left frontal lobe. These electrodes revealed a continuously discharging focus in this region. Craniotomy was repeated at 13 2/12 years with excision of the left supplementary motor region and another focus in the left motor region.

Following this removal, anticonvulsant medication was withdrawn and the patient was free of seizures for seven months. An EEG at 13 4/12 years showed considerable improvement with less activity of the left parietotemporal spike focus. At 13 9/12 years the patient had a further attack in which she became confused and slumped in her chair. Repeat electroencephalography showed a continuous high voltage slow-wave focus in the left parietotemporal region. Dilantin, 100 mg., and Mysoline, 125 mg., were prescribed three times a day. Three months later she had an attack in which her head and eyes turned to the right and in which she was confused and spoke irrationally for a few seconds. The patient had no further seizure till she was 15 6/12 years old, when there was an episode in which she talked in a confused fashion for two hours. Medication was increased to Dilantin, 100 mg. three times a day, and Mysoline, 125 mg. two times a day and 250 mg. q.h.s. She had no further attack in the next six months, the duration of her follow-up.

Comment

The etiology of the epileptogenic lesion or lesions in this patient is not certain. The possibility that the hemiplegia followed a seizure is patent.

The important feature of this case is that it illustrates how the character of the seizure can indicate the localization of the causative lesion, and thus direct persistent surgical intervention following confirmation by direct electrical localization studies.

Special Situations
GENERAL SURGICAL PROCEDURES IN PATIENTS WITH EPILEPSY

The need for an ordinary general surgical operation, such as appendectomy, in a patient with seizures often leads to unwarranted concern on the part of the physician. The fact is that with the simplest precautions there is no special danger in such patients. If an epileptic patient is to undergo general surgery, anticonvulsant medication should be increased to one and one-half times the usual dosage the day before the contemplated surgery. The general anesthesia itself will prevent the complication of a seizure occurring during the operation. However, since anoxemia may precipitate seizures, the patient should be well oxygenated during surgery.

Routine oral anticonvulsant medication should be given postoperatively as soon as feasible. When the patient cannot take medication by mouth for a few days after surgery, anticonvulsant medication should be given parenterally until oral medication can be resumed.

STOPPING ANTICONVULSANT MEDICATION

Anticonvulsant medicines are continued for a period of two to three years after the last seizure. However, the decision as to the duration of continued medication will be influenced by the nature of the patient's occupation and the potential social and economic consequences which might result if the patient had another unexpected seizure. Another important factor to be considered is the approach of adolescence. The onset of puberty in a child who has been free of seizures for two or three years is, nevertheless, a good reason for continuing treatment for at least another year. The findings of follow-up electroencephalographic studies should be another factor influencing the decision to reduce or discontinue medication. If there is much electrographic epileptiform abnormality, it is well to reduce medication much more slowly than otherwise.

If a reduction of medication is to be made, it should be done slowly over a period of four to six months. If the patient is receiving two or more anticonvulsants, they should be discontinued gradually, one at a time. Reducing the drugs individually permits the gradual discontinuation of the least effective member of the combination, and obviates the confusion in the patient's or parents' minds over cutting proportional amounts of two or more drugs. Sudden cessation of medication may precipitate status epilepticus. If seizures recur upon reduction or discontinuation of medication, the previously effective drugs should be reinstituted at the original dosage and maintained for at least a three year period before another attempt to withdraw medication is made. Premature discontinuation or reduction of medication is probably the most common therapeutic mistake. It is often more the fault of the parents than of the physician, because of their eagerness to take the child off medication. Fear of "taking drugs" causing addiction or damage to the patient is a common cause for parents to stop medication, as also are the cost and nuisance of regular drug treatment.

Summary of General Principles in Treatment

The aim of treatment of epilepsy is the control of seizures with as little interference with the life of the patient as possible. This means that the medication should not produce drowsiness or other disturbing side effects, that the patient be able to continue his work and play and that the patient and his family understand that the seizure state is a result of natural causes and that medication can usually control the attacks.

The pattern of seizure often determines the choice of medication, for some anticonvulsant drugs are useful in one type of seizure and may be useless or even precipitate seizures in another kind. It is best to use the most effective drugs first. In generalized or focal seizures, Dilantin, phenobarbital and Mysoline are among the most effective, either individually or in combination. Frequently, only one of these medicines will be required; but each patient presents a different problem, and patients with several types of seizures may require combinations of medications. The best combination of drugs may be found only after much trial.

It is essential to prescribe adequate dosage of a given medication before deciding that the drug is of no value and proceeding to other medications. A frequent cause of failure in the control of seizures is the use of inadequate dosage. This is particularly true with Dilantin and Tridione. It is often necessary to give increasing doses up to toxic level before deciding that a given drug is ineffective.

When two separate drugs are given together, the net anticonvulsant action may be more than the sum of the protective action of each drug individually. Thus it has been found that phenobarbital has a potentiating effect upon the anticonvulsant action of Dilantin, in excess of what would be expected simply from the additive independent effect of the phenobarbital. This property enables one to control seizures at much lower dosage levels than would otherwise be possible.

General health measures are important in epilepsy. Adequate rest and freedom from excessive emotional upset are desirable. Alcohol should be shunned. Constipation may prove a problem since many of the anticonvulsants have a direct, depressant action upon the gut.

In patients who have more seizures at the time of menstruation, Diamox, ammonium chloride and limitation of fluid and salt intake may prove useful.

In general, it is well to tell even youthful patients of their attacks and their nature. Such information is much more likely to be presented in an acceptable way by the physician than by friends or relatives who may have witnessed seizures. The probability of control of these episodes by medication taken faithfully should be emphasized. The parents of an epileptic child should be given as much information as possible about this condition. Some stigma is still attached to epilepsy, and parents are often reassured by the knowledge that the attacks result from the dysfunction of a very small, possibly scarred part of the brain, and not as a result of some supernatural influence. Many are also relieved to learn that epilepsy does not proceed to insanity, and some need reassurance that it is not infectious.

It is good practice to continue medication in full dosage for two to three years after the last seizure. At this time a repeat electroencephalogram should be made, and if this reveals little or no abnormality, the dosage is gradually reduced. If the electroencephalogram reveals significant abnormality, the reduction in medication is postponed or carried out over a more prolonged period. Recurrence of seizures necessitates reinstitution of medication, which is then maintained again at full dosage levels for a further minimum period of three years.

REFERENCES

1. Toman, J. E. P. and Goodman, L. S.: Anticonvulsants. Physiol. Rev., 28: 409, 1948.
2. Toman, J. E. P.: The neuropharmacology of antiepileptics. Electroencephalog. and Clin. Neurophysiol., 1:33, 1949.
3. Forster, F. M.: Medical therapy of epilepsy. Neurology, 1:153, 1951.
4. Abbott, J. A. and Schwab, R. S.: The serious side effects of the newer antiepileptic drugs: their control and prevention. New England J. Med., 242:943, 1950.
5. Moore, M. T.: The treatment of the epileptic individual. J. Albert Einstein Medical Center, 3:12, 1954.
6. Chao, D.: The over-all management of the epileptic child. M. Clin. North America, 42:461, 1958.
7. Merritt, H. H.: Medical treatment in epilepsy. Brit. M. J., 1:666, 1958.

Surgical Treatment of Epilepsy

1. Penfield, W.: The clinical classification of the epilepsies with notes on surgical therapy. Compt. rend. Cong. Neurol. Internat., 3:435, 1949.

2. Meyers, R.: The surgery of "focal" epilepsy: an inquiry into current premises, their implementation and the criteria employed in reporting results. Epilepsia, 3:9, 1954.

3. Falconer, M. A.: Clinical manifestations of temporal lobe epilepsy and their recognition in relation to surgical treatment. Brit. M. J., 2:939, 1954.

4. Penfield, W.: Pitfalls and success in surgical treatment of focal epilepsy. Brit. M. J., 1:669, 1958.

Drug Table

Drug Table

DRUGS	INDICATIONS	DOSAGE 0–1 yr.	5 yr.	12 yr.	16 yr. and up	Mg.–kg. per day	TOXICITY	REMARKS	PREPARATIONS
CELONTIN (methsuximide)	Psychomotor, akinetic and myoclonic seizures; occasionally massive spasms.	75 mg. 2 to 3 times daily.	150 mg. 3 times daily.	300 mg. 2 to 3 times daily.	300 mg. 3 to 5 times daily.	15 to 20.	Drowsiness. Ataxia.	Most useful in psychomotor seizures.	300 mg. capsules.
DEXEDRINE (dextro-amphetamine sulfate)	Absence and akinetic attacks.	1.25 mg. 2 to 3 times daily.	5 mg. 2 times daily.	10 mg. 2 to 3 times daily.	10 mg. 3 to 5 times daily.	0.25 to 0.75.	Restlessness. Irritability. Sleeplessness.	Limited effectiveness. Other amphetamines and mixtures similar.	5 mg. tablets. 1 mg./cc.
DIAMOX (acetazoleamide)	All types of seizures.	125 mg. 3 times daily.	250 mg. 3 times daily.	250 mg. 4 times daily.	250 mg. 4 to 6 times daily.	15 to 90.	Loss of appetite. Acidosis. Numbness of extremities.	Most effective with paroxysmal generalized EEG abnormalities, and with attacks precipitated by overventilation.	250 mg. tablets. 500 mg. amp. I.V. or I.M.
DILANTIN (diphenylhydantoin)	Any seizure with the exception of lapse, myoclonic and akinetic attacks.	20 mg. 3 to 4 times daily.	50 mg. 3 times daily.	100 mg. 3 to 4 times daily.	100 mg. 3 to 6 times daily.	3 to 8.	Gum hypertrophy. Ataxia, diplopia, nystagmus. Rash and fever. Nausea and vomiting. Hirsutism.	The safest and most generally effective anticonvulsant. Only rash and fever are indications for cessation of drug.	30 mg. capsules. 50 mg. Infatabs. 100 mg. capsules. 100 mg. D.A. Kapseals. 25 mg./cc. suspension (i.e., about 1.5 mg. per drop). 250 mg. Steri-Vial with diluent in ampoule.
GEMONIL (metharbital; 5,5-diethyl-1-methyl-barbituric acid)	Massive spasms, myoclonic seizures, etc.	25 mg. 4 to 6 times daily.	50 mg. 4 to 6 times daily.	100 mg. 3 to 4 times daily.	100 mg. 3 to 6 times daily.	5 to 15.	Drowsiness.	Most helpful in the very young.	100 mg. tablets.
MEBARAL (mephobarbital; ethyl methyl phenyl-barbituric acid)	(Same as phenobarbital.)	15 mg. 4 to 5 times daily.	32 mg. 3 to 4 times daily.	100 mg. 3 to 4 times daily.	100 mg. 3 to 6 times daily.	2 to 8.	Drowsiness. Occasional irritability. Rash.	Effective, but may be dulling, though less so than phenobarbital.	32 mg. tablets. 50 mg. tablets. 100 mg. tablets.
MEPROBAMATE (Equanil, Miltown; methyl propyl propanediol dicarbamate)	Absence attacks and convulsive equivalents; occasionally in massive spasms.	200 mg. 2 to 3 times daily.	200 mg. 3 to 5 times daily.	400 mg. 2 to 3 times daily.	400 mg. 3 to 5 times daily.	20 to 40.	Drowsiness. Hyperactivity.	Most effective in subcortical seizures.	200 mg. tablets. 400 mg. tablets.

Drug	Indications	Dosage				Blood level range	Toxic effects	Remarks	How dispensed
MESANTOIN (ethyl methyl phenylhydantoin)	(Same as Dilantin.)	25 mg. 3 to 4 times daily.	50 mg. 3 to 4 times daily.	100 mg. 4 to 6 times daily.	100 mg. 4 to 8 times daily.	4 to 10.	Rash and fever. Leukopenia and agranulocytosis. Ataxia.	Effective, but more frequent toxic reactions than Dilantin.	100 mg. tablets.
MILONTIN (methyl phenylsuccinimide)	Absence, myoclonic, akinetic.	50 mg. 4 to 5 times daily.	250 mg. 3 to 4 times daily.	500 mg. 3 to 6 times daily.	500 mg. 4 to 8 times daily.	20 to 40.	Nephrotoxic (slightly).	Helpful in paroxysmal generalized dysrhythmia.	0.5 gm. capsules. 65 mg./cc. suspension.
MYSOLINE (primidone)	Generalized, focal and psychomotor attacks.	65 mg. 3 to 4 times daily.	250 mg. 2 to 3 times daily.	250 mg. 4 to 6 times daily.	250 mg. 4 to 8 times daily.	12 to 25.	Drowsiness. Ataxia. Skin rash.	Work up dosage slowly. Generally effective.	250 mg. tablets. 65 mg./cc. suspension.
PARADIONE (paramethadione; dimethyl ethyloxazolidinedione)	Lapse and akinetic attacks.	75 mg. 4 to 6 times daily.	150 mg. 4 to 6 times daily.	300 mg. 4 to 6 times daily.	300 mg. 4 to 8 times daily.	20 to 50.	Rash. Leukopenia.	Less effective and less toxic than Tridione.	150 mg. capsules. 300 mg. capsules. 300 mg./cc. elixir.
PARALDEHYDE (paracetaldehyde)	Status attacks. To protect patient during withdrawal of barbiturates or hydantoinates.	1 cc. I.M. 2 cc. R.	3 cc. I.M. 6 cc. R. 4 cc. oral.	2–3 cc. I.V. 5 cc. I.M. 8 cc. oral.	3–4 cc. I.V. 8–20 cc. oral.		Drowsiness. Unpleasant odor.	Much less depression of respiratory center than barbiturates.	Dispensed in bottles and in 5 cc. ampoules.
PHENOBARBITAL (ethyl phenylbarbituric acid)	Any seizure problem.	15 mg. 3 to 4 times daily.	30 mg. 2 to 3 times daily.	60 mg. 2 to 3 times daily.	60 mg. 3 to 4 times daily.	1 to 5.	Drowsiness. Skin rash and fever. Hyperirritability in children.	Effective, but produces dulling.	16 mg. tablets. 32 mg. tablets. 64 mg. tablets. 100 mg. tablets. 4 mg./cc. elixir.
PHENURONE (phenacemide)	Psychomotor attacks (temporal lobe type).	125 mg. 3 to 4 times daily.	250 mg. 4 times daily.	500 mg. 4 times daily.	500 mg. 4 to 6 times daily.	20 to 35.	Hepatotoxic. Leukopenia and agranulocytosis. Rash. Irritability and mental derangement.	Very prone to produce toxic side effects.	0.5 gm. tablets.
TRIDIONE (trimethadione trimethyl oxazolidinedione)	Lapse, myoclonic and akinetic attacks. Other seizures with EEG patterns of 3 per second generalized paroxysmal bursts.	25 mg. 4 to 6 times daily.	150 mg. 4 to 6 times daily.	300 mg. 4 to 6 times daily.	600 mg. 3 to 5 times daily.	20 to 50.	Rash. Leukopenia and agranulocytosis. Photophobia. Irritability.	Often effective in lapse attacks. May be effective in akinetic and myoclonic attacks.	300 mg. capsules. 150 mg. tablets. 37.5 mg./cc. elixir.

Index